Alzheimer's and Dementia

Diet Cookbook and Guide for Seniors

Healthy Brain-Boosting Recipes to Improve Memory and Cognitive Health in Seniors|7 Day Meal Plan

Judy Kelly

Copyright © Judy Kelly, 2024.

All rights reserved. No part of this publication may be reproduced, distributed, or transmitted in any form or by any means, including photocopying, recording, or other electronic or mechanical methods, without the prior written permission of the publisher, except in the case of brief quotations embodied in critical reviews and certain other noncommercial uses permitted by copyright law.

Table of Contents

1. Introduction... 3
2. Chapter 1: The Alzheimer's and Dementia Diet........ 5
3. Chapter 2: Breakfast Recipes..................................... 15
4. Chapter 3: Smoothies and Drinks.............................. 25
5. Chapter 4: Snacks and Appetizers..........................34
6. Chapter 5: Lunch Recipes...43
7. Chapter 6: Dinner Recipes... 55
8. Chapter 7: Side Dishes... 71
9. Chapter 8: Desserts... 82
10. Chapter 9: Meal Plans..92
    - 7-Day Meal Plan...92
    - Tips for Meal Prep and Batch Cooking......................97
11. Chapter 10: Tips for a Healthy Lifestyle.................99
    - Incorporating Physical Activity................................. 99
    - Importance of Social Engagement........................... 101
    - Stress Management Techniques............................. 103
    - Sleep Hygiene for Cognitive Health........................ 105
12. Conclusion... 108

1. Introduction

Welcome to the Alzheimer's and Dementia Diet Cookbook for Seniors. If you or a loved one are navigating the challenges of Alzheimer's or dementia, this book is designed with you in mind. We understand that this journey can be difficult and overwhelming, but it is also filled with moments of love, connection, and hope. Our goal is to support you through this journey by providing nourishing and delicious recipes that promote brain health and cognitive function.

The Importance of Diet in Alzheimer's and Dementia

The connection between diet and brain health is profound. Research has shown that the foods we eat can significantly impact our cognitive abilities, memory, and overall brain function. A well-balanced, nutrient-rich diet can help slow cognitive decline, enhance memory, and improve the quality of life for those living with Alzheimer's and dementia.

This cookbook is more than just a collection of recipes. It is a resource rooted in compassion and understanding, aimed at empowering you to make positive changes that can lead to better brain health. By incorporating these brain-boosting foods into your daily routine, you are taking a proactive step towards supporting cognitive function and overall well-being.

Understanding Brain-Boosting Nutrients

Each recipe in this book has been carefully crafted to include ingredients known for their brain-boosting properties. Foods rich in antioxidants, healthy fats, vitamins, and minerals play a crucial role in maintaining brain health. From vibrant berries and leafy greens to wholesome grains and lean proteins, these recipes are designed to be both delicious and beneficial for your mind.

How to Use This Cookbook

Whether you are a caregiver looking to provide nutritious meals for a loved one, or you are living with Alzheimer's or dementia and seeking to take control of your diet, this cookbook is here to guide you. We've included a variety of recipes to suit different tastes and dietary needs, along with practical tips for meal planning, shopping, and preparation.

We understand that cooking can sometimes feel daunting, especially when dealing with the complexities of Alzheimer's and dementia. That's why we've focused on simple, straightforward recipes that are easy to follow and quick to prepare. Each recipe comes with step-by-step instructions and helpful tips to ensure success in the kitchen, no matter your experience level.

A Journey of Hope and Healing

As you embark on this culinary journey, remember that every small step counts. The path to better brain health is paved with mindful choices, and by choosing to nourish your body with these healthy, brain-boosting recipes, you are making a powerful commitment to your well-being.

This cookbook is dedicated to everyone affected by Alzheimer's and dementia. We hope it brings you comfort, joy, and nourishment, and that it serves as a reminder that you are not alone on this journey. Together, we can create moments of happiness and connection around the dinner table, one meal at a time.

Thank you for allowing us to be a part of your journey. Here's to health, hope, and healing through the power of good food.

2. Chapter 1: The Alzheimer's and Dementia Diet

Key Principles and Guidelines

Maintaining a diet that supports brain health and cognitive function is essential for seniors living with Alzheimer's and dementia. Here are the key principles and guidelines to help you get the most out of your meals and promote overall well-being.

1. Embrace a Mediterranean-Inspired Diet
The Mediterranean diet is renowned for its heart-healthy and brain-boosting properties. It emphasizes:
- Fresh Fruits and Vegetables: Rich in antioxidants, vitamins, and minerals that protect brain cells.
- Whole Grains: Provide sustained energy and essential nutrients for brain function.
- Healthy Fats: Include olive oil, nuts, seeds, and avocados, which are beneficial for brain health.
- Lean Proteins: Opt for fish, poultry, legumes, and plant-based proteins to support cognitive function.

2. Incorporate Brain-Boosting Foods
Certain foods are especially beneficial for brain health:
- Berries: Blueberries, strawberries, and other berries are high in antioxidants that combat oxidative stress and inflammation.
- Leafy Greens: Spinach, kale, and other greens are packed with nutrients like vitamin K, lutein, and folate, which are linked to better cognitive function.
- Nuts and Seeds: Walnuts, almonds, chia seeds, and flaxseeds are excellent sources of omega-3 fatty acids and antioxidants.
- Fatty Fish: Salmon, mackerel, and sardines are rich in omega-3 fatty acids, which are essential for brain health.
- Whole Grains: Brown rice, quinoa, and oatmeal provide fiber and energy without causing spikes in blood sugar levels.

3. Limit Processed Foods and Sugars
- Avoid Refined Sugars and Grains: These can cause inflammation and negatively affect brain function. Opt for natural sweeteners and whole grains instead.
- Minimize Processed Foods: Packaged and processed foods often contain unhealthy fats, high sodium levels, and artificial additives that can harm cognitive health.

4. Stay Hydrated
- Drink Plenty of Water: Dehydration can impair cognitive function and lead to confusion and memory problems. Aim for at least 8 cups of water daily.
- Include Hydrating Foods: Foods like cucumbers, watermelon, and soups can help maintain hydration.

5. Practice Balanced Eating
- Moderation is Key: Balance is crucial. Ensure that your meals include a mix of proteins, healthy fats, and carbohydrates to provide sustained energy and support overall health.
- Portion Control: Be mindful of portion sizes to prevent overeating and maintain a healthy weight.

6. Plan and Prepare Meals in Advance
- Meal Planning: Plan your meals and snacks ahead of time to ensure a balanced diet and reduce the stress of last-minute cooking.
- Batch Cooking: Prepare larger quantities of meals and store portions for later use, making it easier to have healthy options readily available.

7. Encourage Social Eating
- Share Meals: Eating with family and friends can enhance the dining experience, promote social engagement, and provide emotional support.
- Create a Pleasant Environment: Make mealtimes enjoyable and stress-free by setting a calm and inviting table.

8. Tailor to Individual Needs
- Personalize the Diet: Consider individual preferences, dietary restrictions, and specific health conditions when planning meals.
- Monitor and Adjust: Regularly assess the effectiveness of the diet and make necessary adjustments to meet changing needs and preferences.

By following these key principles and guidelines, you can create a diet that not only supports brain health and cognitive function but also enhances the overall quality of life for seniors living with Alzheimer's and dementia. Remember, small changes can make a significant difference, and every meal is an opportunity to nourish the body and mind.

- Foods to Embrace Foods to Embrace

Incorporating the right foods into your diet can significantly impact brain health and cognitive function. Here are the foods you should embrace to support Alzheimer's and dementia care:

1. Berries
- Blueberries, Strawberries, Raspberries, and Blackberries: These are high in antioxidants, particularly flavonoids, which help reduce oxidative stress and inflammation in the brain.

2. Leafy Greens
- Spinach, Kale, Collard Greens, and Swiss Chard: Packed with nutrients such as vitamin K, lutein, folate, and beta-carotene, these greens are known to support brain health and slow cognitive decline.

3. Cruciferous Vegetables
- Broccoli, Cauliflower, Brussels Sprouts, and Cabbage: Rich in antioxidants and glucosinolates, which may reduce the risk of neurodegenerative diseases.

4. Fatty Fish
- Salmon, Mackerel, Sardines, and Trout: These are excellent sources of omega-3 fatty acids, particularly DHA, which is crucial for brain health and function.

5. Nuts and Seeds
- Walnuts, Almonds, Chia Seeds, Flaxseeds, and Pumpkin Seeds: High in healthy fats, antioxidants, and fiber, nuts and seeds support cognitive function and heart health.

6. Whole Grains
- Brown Rice, Quinoa, Oats, Barley, and Whole Wheat: These provide sustained energy and essential nutrients like fiber, vitamins, and minerals, which support overall brain health.

7. Legumes
- Beans, Lentils, Chickpeas, and Peas: Rich in protein, fiber, and vitamins, legumes help maintain stable blood sugar levels and provide sustained energy for the brain.

8. Healthy Fats
- Olive Oil, Avocado, and Coconut Oil: These fats are known for their anti-inflammatory properties and support overall brain health.

9. Fruits
- Oranges, Apples, Bananas, and Grapes: High in vitamins, minerals, and antioxidants, fruits support overall health and cognitive function.

10. Vegetables
- Carrots, Sweet Potatoes, Bell Peppers, and Squash: Rich in vitamins, minerals, and antioxidants, these vegetables promote brain health and reduce inflammation.

11. Herbs and Spices
- Turmeric, Cinnamon, Sage, and Rosemary: Known for their anti-inflammatory and antioxidant properties, these can enhance brain function and memory.

12. Dairy and Alternatives
- Greek Yogurt, Kefir, and Plant-Based Milks: These provide essential nutrients like calcium, vitamin D, and probiotics, which support overall health.

13. Lean Proteins
- Chicken, Turkey, Tofu, and Tempeh: These are important for maintaining muscle mass and providing sustained energy.

14. Hydrating Foods
- Cucumbers, Watermelon, and Citrus Fruits: These help maintain hydration, which is crucial for cognitive function and overall health.

15. Herbal Teas
- Green Tea, Chamomile, and Peppermint Tea: These are rich in antioxidants and can promote relaxation and mental clarity.

By incorporating these foods into your daily diet, you can create meals that are not only delicious but also beneficial for brain health and cognitive function. These foods provide the essential nutrients needed to support overall well-being and improve the quality of life for those living with Alzheimer's and dementia.

- **Foods to Avoid Foods to Avoid**

To support brain health and reduce the risk of cognitive decline, it is important to limit or avoid certain foods that can negatively impact brain function and overall well-being. Here are the foods you should be cautious about:

1. Refined Sugars and Sweets
- Sugary Snacks and Desserts: Cookies, cakes, candy, and pastries can cause spikes in blood sugar levels, leading to inflammation and negatively affecting brain health.
- Sugary Beverages: Sodas, energy drinks, and sweetened teas are high in added sugars, which can contribute to cognitive decline and other health issues.

2. Processed Foods
- Packaged Snacks: Chips, crackers, and other processed snacks often contain unhealthy fats, high sodium, and artificial additives.
- Pre-Packaged Meals: Frozen dinners, instant noodles, and other convenience foods can be high in unhealthy fats, sodium, and preservatives.

3. Trans Fats
- Hydrogenated Oils: Found in margarine, shortening, and some baked goods, trans fats are linked to inflammation and an increased risk of neurodegenerative diseases.
- Fried Foods: French fries, fried chicken, and other deep-fried foods often contain trans fats and unhealthy oils.

4. Saturated Fats
- Fatty Meats: Bacon, sausage, and other high-fat meats can increase cholesterol levels and negatively impact brain health.
- Full-Fat Dairy Products: Whole milk, cream, and certain cheeses should be consumed in moderation due to their high saturated fat content.

5. High-Sodium Foods
- Processed Meats: Ham, salami, and other processed meats are often high in sodium, which can contribute to high blood pressure and increase the risk of stroke and cognitive decline.
- Salty Snacks: Pretzels, salted nuts, and other salty snacks can lead to excessive sodium intake.

6. Artificial Additives and Preservatives
- Artificial Sweeteners: Aspartame, saccharin, and other artificial sweeteners can have negative effects on brain health and cognitive function.
- Food Dyes and Additives: Many processed foods contain artificial colors and preservatives that can be harmful to overall health.

7. Alcohol
- Excessive Alcohol Consumption: Drinking large amounts of alcohol can impair brain function, memory, and cognitive abilities. Moderate alcohol consumption, particularly red wine, is generally considered acceptable, but it should be approached with caution.

8. High-Glycemic Index Foods
- Refined Carbohydrates: White bread, white rice, and other refined grains can cause rapid spikes in blood sugar levels, leading to inflammation and cognitive decline.
- Sugary Breakfast Cereals: Many cereals are high in added sugars and refined grains, making them a poor choice for brain health.

9. Fast Food
- Burgers, Hot Dogs, and Fast-Food Meals: These often contain unhealthy fats, high sodium levels, and low nutritional value, which can negatively affect brain health.

10. Highly Processed Cooking Oils
- Vegetable Oils: Corn oil, soybean oil, and other highly processed vegetable oils can be high in omega-6 fatty acids, which can promote inflammation if consumed in excess.

By avoiding or limiting these foods, you can help reduce inflammation, support brain health, and improve overall well-being. Focus on whole, nutrient-dense foods that provide the essential nutrients needed for optimal cognitive function and a healthier life.

- Meal Planning Tips

Meal planning is an essential tool for maintaining a nutritious diet that supports brain health and cognitive function for seniors with Alzheimer's and dementia. Here are some practical tips to help you effectively plan meals:

1. Set Realistic Goals
- Start Simple: Begin with a few days of meal planning at a time to avoid feeling overwhelmed.
- Plan Balanced Meals: Include a variety of foods from different food groups to ensure nutritional adequacy.

2. Consider Individual Preferences and Needs
- Consult with a Dietitian: If possible, seek advice from a healthcare professional or dietitian who specializes in senior nutrition and cognitive health.
- Take Preferences into Account: Incorporate foods and flavors that are familiar and enjoyable for the person with Alzheimer's or dementia.

3. Create a Weekly Menu
- Use a Planner: Write down your meal ideas for the week, including breakfast, lunch, dinner, and snacks.
- Rotate Recipes: Include a mix of favorite recipes and new dishes to keep meals interesting.

4. Focus on Nutrient-Dense Foods
- Include Brain-Boosting Foods: Plan meals that incorporate berries, leafy greens, fatty fish, nuts, whole grains, and other foods known for their cognitive benefits.
- Variety is Key: Aim for a rainbow of colors on your plate to ensure a diverse range of nutrients.

5. Plan for Regular Meals and Snacks
- Establish Routine: Consistent mealtimes can help regulate appetite and promote better digestion.

- Healthy Snacking: Prepare nutritious snacks like fresh fruit, yogurt, nuts, or homemade energy bars for between-meal munching.

6. Consider Practicality and Convenience
- Batch Cooking: Prepare larger batches of soups, stews, or casseroles that can be portioned and frozen for later use.
- Quick and Easy Options: Include simple recipes that require minimal preparation time, especially for busy days.

7. Make Use of Leftovers
- Plan Double Portions: Cook extra portions of meals that can be enjoyed as leftovers for the next day's lunch or dinner.
- Repurpose Ingredients: Use leftover roasted vegetables in salads or sandwiches for a quick meal option.

8. Shop Wisely
- Prepare a List: Before shopping, make a list of ingredients needed for your planned meals to avoid impulse purchases.
- Stick to the Perimeter: Focus on fresh produce, lean proteins, dairy, and whole grains found around the perimeter of the grocery store.

9. Adapt and Modify as Needed
- Be Flexible: Adjust your meal plan based on changes in preferences, appetite, or dietary requirements.
- Monitor Effectiveness: Keep track of how meals are received and adjust recipes or portions accordingly.

10. Seek Support and Share Responsibilities
- Involve Others: Share meal planning responsibilities with family members, caregivers, or friends to lighten the load.
- Mealtime Support: Offer assistance as needed during meal preparation and dining to ensure a positive and enjoyable experience.

By implementing these meal planning tips, you can create a supportive and nourishing diet that enhances brain health and overall well-being for seniors living with Alzheimer's and dementia. Remember, the goal is to provide enjoyable meals that contribute to a higher quality of life through nutritious eating habits.

3. Chapter 2: Breakfast Recipes

1. Berry-Almond Overnight Oats

Ingredients:
- 1/2 cup rolled oats
- 1/2 cup almond milk
- 1/4 cup Greek yogurt
- 1/4 cup mixed berries (blueberries, strawberries)
- 1 tbsp chia seeds
- 1 tbsp almond butter
- 1 tsp honey or maple syrup (optional)

Instructions:
1. In a bowl or jar, combine oats, almond milk, Greek yogurt, chia seeds, and almond butter.
2. Stir well to mix ingredients thoroughly.
3. Cover and refrigerate overnight.
4. In the morning, top with mixed berries and drizzle with honey or maple syrup if desired. Serve chilled.

2. Spinach and Feta Egg Muffins

Ingredients:
- 6 eggs
- 1/2 cup spinach, chopped
- 1/4 cup feta cheese, crumbled
- 1/4 cup red bell pepper, diced
- Salt and pepper to taste
- Cooking spray or olive oil for greasing

Instructions:
1. Preheat oven to 350°F (175°C). Grease a muffin tin with cooking spray or olive oil.
2. In a bowl, whisk together eggs, spinach, feta cheese, red bell pepper, salt, and pepper.
3. Pour egg mixture evenly into muffin cups, filling each about 3/4 full.

4. Bake for 20-25 minutes, or until eggs are set and muffins are lightly browned on top.
5. Remove from oven and let cool slightly before serving.

3. Avocado Toast with Smoked Salmon
Ingredients:
- 2 slices whole wheat or gluten-free bread, toasted
- 1 ripe avocado
- Juice of 1/2 lemon
- Salt and pepper to taste
- 2 oz smoked salmon
- Fresh dill or chives for garnish

Instructions:
1. Mash avocado in a bowl and mix with lemon juice, salt, and pepper.
2. Spread avocado mixture evenly on toasted bread slices.
3. Top with smoked salmon and garnish with fresh dill or chives.
4. Serve immediately.

4. Greek Yogurt Parfait
Ingredients:
- 1 cup Greek yogurt
- 1/2 cup mixed berries (blueberries, strawberries)
- 1/4 cup granola or oats
- 1 tbsp honey or maple syrup (optional)

Instructions:
1. In a glass or bowl, layer Greek yogurt, mixed berries, and granola or oats.
2. Repeat layers as desired.
3. Drizzle with honey or maple syrup if desired.
4. Serve chilled.

5. Banana Nut Smoothie
Ingredients:
- 1 ripe banana

- 1/2 cup Greek yogurt
- 1/2 cup almond milk
- 1 tbsp almond butter
- 1 tbsp honey or maple syrup (optional)
- 1/4 cup walnuts, chopped

Instructions:
1. In a blender, combine banana, Greek yogurt, almond milk, almond butter, and honey or maple syrup.
2. Blend until smooth.
3. Pour into a glass and top with chopped walnuts.
4. Serve immediately.

6. Veggie and Cheese Omelette

Ingredients:
- 2 eggs
- 1/4 cup mixed vegetables (bell peppers, spinach, tomatoes), chopped
- 1/4 cup shredded cheddar cheese
- Salt and pepper to taste
- Cooking spray or olive oil for greasing

Instructions:
1. In a bowl, whisk together eggs, mixed vegetables, shredded cheese, salt, and pepper.
2. Heat a non-stick skillet over medium heat and lightly grease with cooking spray or olive oil.
3. Pour egg mixture into the skillet, spreading evenly.
4. Cook for 2-3 minutes, then flip and cook for an additional 2-3 minutes, until eggs are fully cooked and cheese is melted.
5. Slide omelette onto a plate and serve hot.

7. Blueberry Quinoa Breakfast Bowl

Ingredients:
- 1/2 cup cooked quinoa
- 1/4 cup almond milk

- 1/2 cup fresh blueberries
- 1 tbsp honey or maple syrup (optional)
- 1 tbsp sliced almonds

Instructions:
1. In a bowl, combine cooked quinoa and almond milk.
2. Top with fresh blueberries, honey or maple syrup (if using), and sliced almonds.
3. Serve warm or chilled.

8. Apple Cinnamon Baked Oatmeal

Ingredients:
- 1 cup rolled oats
- 1 cup almond milk
- 1 apple, peeled and diced
- 1 tbsp maple syrup
- 1 tsp cinnamon
- 1/4 cup chopped nuts (walnuts or almonds)

Instructions:
1. Preheat oven to 350°F (175°C). Grease a baking dish with cooking spray or olive oil.
2. In a bowl, mix together rolled oats, almond milk, diced apple, maple syrup, cinnamon, and chopped nuts.
3. Pour mixture into the baking dish and spread evenly.
4. Bake for 25-30 minutes, or until oats are cooked and top is golden brown.
5. Remove from oven and let cool slightly before serving.

9. Chia Seed Pudding

Ingredients:
- 1/4 cup chia seeds
- 1 cup almond milk
- 1 tbsp honey or maple syrup
- 1/2 tsp vanilla extract

- Fresh berries for topping

Instructions:
1. In a bowl or jar, mix together chia seeds, almond milk, honey or maple syrup, and vanilla extract.
2. Stir well to combine.
3. Cover and refrigerate for at least 2 hours or overnight, until mixture thickens and becomes pudding-like.
4. Top with fresh berries before serving.

10. Spinach and Mushroom Breakfast Quesadilla
Ingredients:
- 2 whole wheat or gluten-free tortillas
- 1 cup fresh spinach
- 1/2 cup mushrooms, sliced
- 1/4 cup shredded mozzarella cheese
- Salt and pepper to taste
- Cooking spray or olive oil for greasing

Instructions:
1. Heat a non-stick skillet over medium heat and lightly grease with cooking spray or olive oil.
2. Place one tortilla in the skillet and top with spinach, mushrooms, shredded mozzarella cheese, salt, and pepper.
3. Place the second tortilla on top and press down gently.
4. Cook for 2-3 minutes on each side, or until tortilla is golden brown and cheese is melted.
5. Remove from skillet, slice into wedges, and serve hot.

11. Peanut Butter Banana Toast
Ingredients:
- 2 slices whole wheat or gluten-free bread, toasted
- 2 tbsp peanut butter
- 1 banana, sliced
- 1 tbsp honey or maple syrup (optional)

Instructions:
1. Spread peanut butter evenly on toasted bread slices.
2. Top with sliced banana.
3. Drizzle with honey or maple syrup if desired.
4. Serve immediately.

12. Veggie Breakfast Burrito

Ingredients:
- 1 whole wheat or gluten-free tortilla
- 2 eggs, scrambled
- 1/4 cup black beans, drained and rinsed
- 1/4 cup diced tomatoes
- 1/4 cup diced avocado
- Fresh cilantro for garnish
- Salsa or hot sauce (optional)

Instructions:
1. Heat tortilla in a skillet or microwave until warm.
2. Fill tortilla with scrambled eggs, black beans, diced tomatoes, and diced avocado.
3. Roll up tortilla and garnish with fresh cilantro.
4. Serve with salsa or hot sauce on the side if desired.

13. Greek Yogurt Pancakes

Ingredients:
- 1 cup Greek yogurt
- 2 eggs
- 1/2 cup whole wheat flour
- 1 tsp baking powder
- 1/2 tsp vanilla extract
- Fresh berries for topping
- Maple syrup for drizzling

Instructions:
1. In a bowl, whisk together Greek yogurt, eggs, whole wheat flour, baking powder, and vanilla extract until smooth.
2. Heat a non-stick skillet or griddle over medium heat.
3. Pour batter onto the skillet to form pancakes.
4. Cook for 2-3 minutes on each side, or until pancakes are golden brown and cooked through.
5. Top with fresh berries and drizzle with maple syrup before serving.

14. Cottage Cheese with Fresh Fruit

Ingredients:
- 1/2 cup cottage cheese
- 1/2 cup mixed fresh fruit (berries, kiwi, mango)
- 1 tbsp honey or maple syrup (optional)
- 1 tbsp chopped nuts (walnuts or almonds)

Instructions:
1. Spoon cottage cheese into a bowl.
2. Top with mixed fresh fruit.
3. Drizzle with honey or maple syrup if desired.
4. Sprinkle with chopped nuts before serving.

15. Mediterranean Veggie Breakfast Bowl

Ingredients:
- 1/2 cup cooked quinoa or brown rice
- 1/4 cup hummus
- 1/4 cup cherry tomatoes, halved
- 1/4 cup cucumber, diced- 1/4 cup bell pepper, diced
- 1/4 cup Kalamata olives, sliced
- 1/4 cup feta cheese, crumbled
- Fresh parsley for garnish
- Lemon wedges for serving

Instructions:
1. In a bowl, layer cooked quinoa or brown rice at the bottom.

2. Arrange hummus, cherry tomatoes, cucumber, bell pepper, and Kalamata olives on top.
3. Sprinkle with crumbled feta cheese and garnish with fresh parsley.
4. Serve with lemon wedges on the side for squeezing over the bowl.

16. Almond Butter Banana Smoothie Bowl

Ingredients:
- 1 ripe banana, frozen
- 1/4 cup almond butter
- 1/2 cup almond milk
- 1 tbsp honey or maple syrup (optional)
- Toppings: sliced banana, granola, chia seeds, shredded coconut

Instructions:
1. In a blender, combine frozen banana, almond butter, almond milk, and honey or maple syrup.
2. Blend until smooth and creamy.
3. Pour into a bowl and top with sliced banana, granola, chia seeds, and shredded coconut.
4. Serve immediately.

17. Tomato Basil Mozzarella Breakfast Sandwich

Ingredients:
- 2 slices whole grain bread, toasted
- 1/4 cup fresh mozzarella, sliced
- 1/4 cup cherry tomatoes, sliced
- Fresh basil leaves
- Balsamic glaze (optional)
- Olive oil for drizzling

Instructions:
1. Layer fresh mozzarella slices on one slice of toasted bread.
2. Top with sliced cherry tomatoes and fresh basil leaves.
3. Drizzle with balsamic glaze and olive oil.
4. Place the second slice of toasted bread on top.

5. Slice sandwich in half and serve immediately.

18. Pumpkin Spice Chia Pudding
Ingredients:
- 1/4 cup chia seeds
- 1 cup almond milk
- 1/4 cup pumpkin puree
- 1 tbsp maple syrup
- 1/2 tsp pumpkin pie spice
- Pumpkin seeds for topping

Instructions:
1. In a bowl or jar, mix together chia seeds, almond milk, pumpkin puree, maple syrup, and pumpkin pie spice.
2. Stir well to combine.
3. Cover and refrigerate for at least 2 hours or overnight, until mixture thickens.
4. Top with pumpkin seeds before serving.

19. Mediterranean Egg White Scramble
Ingredients:
- 4 egg whites
- 1/4 cup cherry tomatoes, halved
- 1/4 cup spinach, chopped
- 1/4 cup black olives, sliced
- 1/4 cup feta cheese, crumbled
- Salt and pepper to taste
- Cooking spray or olive oil for greasing

Instructions:
1. Heat a non-stick skillet over medium heat and lightly grease with cooking spray or olive oil.
2. Add cherry tomatoes, spinach, and black olives to the skillet. Cook for 2-3 minutes, until vegetables are tender.
3. Pour in egg whites and cook, stirring gently, until eggs are set.

4. Season with salt and pepper to taste.
5. Sprinkle with crumbled feta cheese before serving.

20. Almond Flour Pancakes

Ingredients:
- 1 cup almond flour
- 2 eggs
- 1/2 cup almond milk
- 1 tbsp maple syrup
- 1/2 tsp baking powder
- 1/2 tsp vanilla extract
- Fresh berries for topping

Instructions:
1. In a bowl, whisk together almond flour, eggs, almond milk, maple syrup, baking powder, and vanilla extract until smooth.
2. Heat a non-stick skillet or griddle over medium heat.
3. Pour batter onto the skillet to form pancakes.
4. Cook for 2-3 minutes on each side, or until pancakes are golden brown and cooked through.
5. Top with fresh berries before serving.

4. Chapter 3: Smoothies and Drinks

1. Berry Blast Smoothie

Ingredients:
- 1/2 cup mixed berries (blueberries, strawberries, raspberries)
- 1/2 banana, frozen
- 1/2 cup Greek yogurt
- 1/2 cup almond milk
- 1 tbsp honey or maple syrup (optional)
- Ice cubes (optional)

Instructions:
1. Combine mixed berries, frozen banana, Greek yogurt, almond milk, and honey or maple syrup in a blender.
2. Blend until smooth.
3. Add ice cubes if desired and blend again until desired consistency is reached.
4. Pour into a glass and serve immediately.

2. Green Goodness Smoothie

Ingredients:
- 1 cup spinach
- 1/2 cup kale
- 1/2 cucumber, peeled and chopped
- 1/2 avocado, peeled and pitted
- 1/2 cup pineapple chunks
- 1/2 cup coconut water or almond milk

Instructions:
1. Place spinach, kale, cucumber, avocado, and pineapple chunks in a blender.
2. Add coconut water or almond milk.
3. Blend until smooth and creamy.
4. Pour into a glass and serve chilled.

3. Tropical Turmeric Smoothie

Ingredients:
- 1/2 cup mango chunks
- 1/2 cup pineapple chunks
- 1 banana, frozen
- 1/2 tsp turmeric powder
- 1/2 cup Greek yogurt
- 1/2 cup coconut water or almond milk

Instructions:
1. Combine mango chunks, pineapple chunks, frozen banana, turmeric powder, Greek yogurt, and coconut water or almond milk in a blender.
2. Blend until smooth and creamy.
3. Pour into a glass and serve immediately.

4. Coconut Water with Mint and Lime

Ingredients:
- 1 cup coconut water
- Fresh mint leaves
- Lime slices

Instructions:
1. Fill a glass with coconut water.
2. Add fresh mint leaves and lime slices.
3. Stir gently and let sit for a few minutes to infuse flavors.
4. Serve chilled.

5. Ginger Lemonade

Ingredients:
- 1 cup water
- Juice of 1 lemon
- 1 tbsp honey or maple syrup (optional)
- 1/2 inch piece of ginger, grated
- Ice cubes

Instructions:
1. In a glass, combine water, lemon juice, honey or maple syrup (if using), and grated ginger.
2. Stir well until honey or maple syrup is dissolved.
3. Add ice cubes and stir again.
4. Serve chilled.

6. Herbal Iced Tea

Ingredients:
- 2 cups water
- 2 tsp herbal tea (such as chamomile, peppermint, or hibiscus)
- Fresh lemon slices
- Fresh mint leaves
- Honey or maple syrup to taste (optional)

Instructions:
1. Bring water to a boil in a saucepan.
2. Remove from heat and add herbal tea.
3. Let steep for 5-7 minutes, then strain into a pitcher.
4. Let cool to room temperature, then refrigerate until chilled.
5. Serve over ice with fresh lemon slices, mint leaves, and sweeten with honey or maple syrup if desired.

7. Blueberry Avocado Smoothie

Ingredients:
- 1/2 cup blueberries
- 1/2 avocado, peeled and pitted
- 1/2 cup spinach
- 1/2 cup almond milk or coconut water
- 1 tbsp honey or maple syrup (optional)
- Ice cubes (optional)

Instructions:
1. Combine blueberries, avocado, spinach, almond milk or coconut water, and honey or maple syrup in a blender.

2. Blend until smooth and creamy.
3. Add ice cubes if desired and blend again until desired consistency is reached.
4. Pour into a glass and serve immediately.

8. Banana Almond Butter Smoothie
Ingredients:
- 1 banana
- 2 tbsp almond butter
- 1/2 cup Greek yogurt
- 1/2 cup almond milk
- 1 tbsp honey or maple syrup (optional)
- Ice cubes (optional)

Instructions:
1. Place banana, almond butter, Greek yogurt, almond milk, and honey or maple syrup in a blender.
2. Blend until smooth.
3. Add ice cubes if desired and blend again until smooth and creamy.
4. Pour into a glass and serve chilled.

9. Kale Pineapple Smoothie
Ingredients:
- 1 cup kale, chopped
- 1 cup pineapple chunks
- 1/2 cup cucumber, chopped
- Juice of 1/2 lime
- 1/2 cup coconut water or almond milk
- Ice cubes (optional)

Instructions:
1. Combine kale, pineapple chunks, cucumber, lime juice, and coconut water or almond milk in a blender.
2. Blend until smooth and creamy.

3. Add ice cubes if desired and blend again until desired consistency is reached.
4. Pour into a glass and serve immediately.

10. Berry Hibiscus Iced Tea

Ingredients:
- 2 cups water
- 2 tsp dried hibiscus flowers
- 1/2 cup mixed berries (strawberries, raspberries)
- Fresh lemon slices
- Honey or maple syrup to taste (optional)

Instructions:
1. Bring water to a boil in a saucepan.
2. Remove from heat and add dried hibiscus flowers.
3. Let steep for 10-15 minutes, then strain into a pitcher.
4. Let cool to room temperature, then refrigerate until chilled.
5. Serve over ice with mixed berries, fresh lemon slices, and sweeten with honey or maple syrup if desired.

11. Mango Lassi

Ingredients:
- 1 cup ripe mango, diced
- 1/2 cup Greek yogurt
- 1/2 cup almond milk or coconut milk
- 1 tbsp honey or maple syrup (optional)
- Pinch of cardamom powder (optional)
- Ice cubes (optional)

Instructions:
1. Place diced mango, Greek yogurt, almond milk or coconut milk, honey or maple syrup, and cardamom powder in a blender.
2. Blend until smooth and creamy.
3. Add ice cubes if desired and blend again until smooth.
4. Pour into a glass and serve chilled.

12. Watermelon Mint Cooler

Ingredients:
- 2 cups watermelon, diced
- Juice of 1/2 lime
- Fresh mint leaves
- Sparkling water or plain water
- Ice cubes

Instructions:
1. In a blender, combine diced watermelon and lime juice.
2. Blend until smooth.
3. Fill glasses with ice cubes and pour watermelon mixture over the ice.
4. Top with sparkling water or plain water.
5. Garnish with fresh mint leaves and serve immediately.

13. Strawberry Banana Spinach Smoothie

Ingredients:
- 1 cup strawberries, hulled
- 1 banana
- 1 cup spinach
- 1/2 cup Greek yogurt
- 1/2 cup almond milk or coconut water
- Ice cubes (optional)

Instructions:
1. Combine strawberries, banana, spinach, Greek yogurt, and almond milk or coconut water in a blender.
2. Blend until smooth and creamy.
3. Add ice cubes if desired and blend again until desired consistency is reached.
4. Pour into a glass and serve immediately.

14. Peanut Butter Chocolate Smoothie

Ingredients:
- 1 banana, frozen

- 2 tbsp peanut butter
- 1 tbsp cocoa powder
- 1/2 cup almond milk or coconut milk
- 1 tbsp honey or maple syrup (optional)
- Ice cubes (optional)

Instructions:
1. In a blender, combine frozen banana, peanut butter, cocoa powder, almond milk or coconut milk, and honey or maple syrup.
2. Blend until smooth and creamy.
3. Add ice cubes if desired and blend again until smooth.
4. Pour into a glass and serve chilled.

15. Beetroot Berry Smoothie

Ingredients:
- 1 small beetroot, cooked and peeled
- 1/2 cup mixed berries (blueberries, raspberries)
- 1/2 cup Greek yogurt
- 1/2 cup almond milk or coconut water
- 1 tbsp honey or maple syrup (optional)
- Ice cubes (optional)

Instructions:
1. Cut cooked and peeled beetroot into chunks.
2. Combine beetroot chunks, mixed berries, Greek yogurt, almond milk or coconut water, and honey or maple syrup in a blender.
3. Blend until smooth and creamy.
4. Add ice cubes if desired and blend again until desired consistency is reached.
5. Pour into a glass and serve immediately.

16. Apple Ginger Detox Water

Ingredients:
- 1 apple, thinly sliced
- 1-inch piece of ginger, thinly sliced

- Fresh mint leaves
- Water

Instructions:
1. In a pitcher, combine apple slices, ginger slices, and fresh mint leaves.
2. Fill the pitcher with water.
3. Refrigerate for at least 1 hour to allow flavors to infuse.
4. Serve chilled, with ice cubes if desired.

17. Cucumber Mint Infused Water
Ingredients:
- 1/2 cucumber, thinly sliced
- Fresh mint leaves
- Water

Instructions:
1. In a pitcher, combine cucumber slices and fresh mint leaves.
2. Fill the pitcher with water.
3. Refrigerate for at least 1 hour to allow flavors to infuse.
4. Serve chilled, with ice cubes if desired.

18. Golden Milk Latte
Ingredients:
- 1 cup almond milk or coconut milk
- 1/2 tsp ground turmeric
- 1/4 tsp ground cinnamon
- Pinch of ground ginger
- Pinch of ground black pepper
- 1 tsp honey or maple syrup (optional)

Instructions:
1. In a small saucepan, heat almond milk or coconut milk over medium heat.
2. Stir in ground turmeric, ground cinnamon, ground ginger, and ground black pepper.

3. Whisk continuously until mixture is hot but not boiling.
4. Remove from heat and stir in honey or maple syrup if desired.
5. Pour into a mug and serve warm.

19. Citrus Green Tea

Ingredients:
- 2 cups water
- 1 green tea bag
- Juice of 1/2 lemon
- Juice of 1/2 orange
- Honey or maple syrup to taste (optional)
- Ice cubes

Instructions:
1. Bring water to a boil in a saucepan.
2. Remove from heat and add green tea bag.
3. Let steep for 3-5 minutes, then remove tea bag.
4. Let cool to room temperature.
5. Stir in lemon juice, orange juice, and honey or maple syrup if desired.
6. Serve over ice cubes.

20. Carrot Apple Ginger Juice

Ingredients:
- 2 carrots, peeled and chopped
- 1 apple, cored and chopped
- 1-inch piece of ginger, peeled
- Water (optional)

Instructions:
1. In a juicer, process carrots, apple, and ginger until juiced.
2. If the juice is too thick, add a little water to reach desired consistency.
3. Pour into a glass and serve immediately.

5. Chapter 4: Snacks and Appetizers

1. Greek Yogurt with Berries

Ingredients:
- 1/2 cup Greek yogurt
- Handful of mixed berries (blueberries, strawberries, raspberries)
- Drizzle of honey or maple syrup (optional)

Instructions:
1. Spoon Greek yogurt into a bowl.
2. Top with mixed berries.
3. Drizzle with honey or maple syrup if desired.
4. Serve immediately.

2. Nut Butter Apple Slices

Ingredients:
- 1 apple, sliced
- Nut butter of choice (almond butter, peanut butter)
- Optional toppings: chia seeds, granola

Instructions:
1. Slice apple into thin rounds or wedges.
2. Spread nut butter on apple slices.
3. Sprinkle with optional toppings like chia seeds or granola.
4. Serve immediately.

3. Veggie Sticks with Hummus

Ingredients:
- Assorted vegetable sticks (carrots, cucumbers, bell peppers)
- Hummus for dipping

Instructions:
1. Wash and cut vegetables into sticks.
2. Serve with hummus for dipping.
3. Arrange on a plate for easy access.

4. Caprese Salad Skewers
Ingredients:
- Cherry tomatoes
- Fresh mozzarella balls
- Fresh basil leaves
- Balsamic glaze

Instructions:
1. Thread cherry tomatoes, fresh mozzarella balls, and basil leaves onto skewers.
2. Arrange on a serving platter.
3. Drizzle with balsamic glaze before serving.

5. Smoked Salmon Cucumber Bites
Ingredients:
- English cucumber, sliced into rounds
- Smoked salmon slices
- Cream cheese or Greek yogurt
- Fresh dill or chives for garnish

Instructions:
1. Spread a small amount of cream cheese or Greek yogurt on each cucumber round.
2. Top with smoked salmon slices.
3. Garnish with fresh dill or chives.
4. Serve chilled.

6. Avocado Tuna Salad Cups
Ingredients:
- Avocado, halved and pitted
- Canned tuna, drained
- Lemon juice
- Salt and pepper to taste
- Optional: diced celery, red onion, or capers

Instructions:
1. Scoop out some avocado flesh to create a larger cavity.
2. In a bowl, mix tuna with lemon juice, salt, pepper, and optional ingredients if using.
3. Spoon tuna mixture into avocado halves.
4. Serve immediately.

7. Trail Mix

Ingredients:
- Mixed nuts (almonds, walnuts, cashews)
- Dried fruits (raisins, cranberries, apricots)
- Dark chocolate chips or chunks

Instructions:
1. Combine mixed nuts, dried fruits, and dark chocolate chips or chunks in a bowl.
2. Mix well.
3. Portion into small containers or snack bags for easy grab-and-go.

8. Cheese and Crackers Plate

Ingredients:
- Assorted cheese slices or cubes (cheddar, Swiss, gouda)
- Whole grain crackers
- Grapes or apple slices

Instructions:
1. Arrange cheese slices or cubes on a plate.
2. Serve with whole grain crackers and fresh fruit slices.
3. Provide a small knife for easier serving if needed.

9. Smoothie Bowl

Ingredients:
- Smoothie of choice (such as the Berry Blast or Green Goodness smoothie from earlier)
- Toppings: Fresh berries, granola, chia seeds, coconut flakes

Instructions:
1. Prepare a smoothie of choice and pour into a bowl.
2. Top with fresh berries, granola, chia seeds, and coconut flakes.
3. Serve immediately with a spoon.

10. Stuffed Bell Peppers

Ingredients:
- Mini bell peppers, halved and seeded
- Cream cheese or goat cheese
- Fresh herbs (parsley, chives)
- Optional: diced vegetables (tomatoes, cucumbers)

Instructions:
1. Fill mini bell pepper halves with cream cheese or goat cheese.
2. Garnish with fresh herbs and optional diced vegetables.
3. Arrange on a serving platter and serve chilled.

11. Spinach Artichoke Dip with Veggie Crudites

Ingredients:
- Spinach artichoke dip (store-bought or homemade)
- Assorted vegetable sticks (carrots, celery, bell peppers)

Instructions:
1. Place spinach artichoke dip in a serving bowl.
2. Arrange vegetable sticks around the dip bowl.
3. Serve immediately for dipping.

12. Cucumber Avocado Sushi Rolls

Ingredients:
- English cucumber, thinly sliced lengthwise
- Avocado slices
- Smoked salmon or cooked shrimp (optional)
- Sushi rice
- Nori sheets

Instructions:
1. Lay a nori sheet flat on a bamboo sushi mat or clean surface.
2. Spread a thin layer of sushi rice over the nori sheet.
3. Arrange cucumber slices, avocado slices, and optional smoked salmon or shrimp on top of the rice.
4. Roll the nori sheet tightly using the bamboo mat.
5. Slice into bite-sized pieces and serve chilled.

13. Fruit Salad Cups

Ingredients:
- Assorted fresh fruits (berries, melons, grapes)
- Greek yogurt or cottage cheese
- Optional: honey or maple syrup

Instructions:
1. Chop fresh fruits into bite-sized pieces.
2. Spoon Greek yogurt or cottage cheese into small bowls or cups.
3. Top with chopped fruits.
4. Drizzle with honey or maple syrup if desired.
5. Serve chilled.

14. Mini Quiches

Ingredients:
- Store-bought or homemade mini quiche (spinach, mushroom, or ham)
- Fresh herbs for garnish

Instructions:
1. Heat mini quiches according to package instructions if store-bought.
2. Arrange on a serving platter.
3. Garnish with fresh herbs before serving.

15. Rice Cake Toppings

Ingredients:
- Rice cakes

- Toppings: Peanut butter, almond butter, sliced banana, honey or maple syrup

Instructions:
1. Spread peanut butter or almond butter on rice cakes.
2. Top with sliced banana.
3. Drizzle with honey or maple syrup.
4. Serve immediately.

16. Bruschetta with Tomato and Basil
Ingredients:
- Baguette, sliced and toasted
- Cherry tomatoes, diced
- Fresh basil leaves, chopped
- Olive oil
- Balsamic glaze

Instructions:
1. Brush baguette slices with olive oil and toast until golden brown.
2. In a bowl, mix diced cherry tomatoes and chopped basil.
3. Spoon tomato mixture onto toasted baguette slices.
4. Drizzle with balsamic glaze before serving.

17. Mediterranean Veggie Platter
Ingredients:
- Assorted olives
- Cherry tomatoes
- Cucumber slices
- Hummus or tzatziki for dipping
- Pita bread or crackers

Instructions:
1. Arrange assorted olives, cherry tomatoes, and cucumber slices on a platter.
2. Serve with hummus or tzatziki for dipping.

3. Provide pita bread or crackers on the side.

18. Cheese Quesadilla Triangles

Ingredients:
- Flour tortillas
- Shredded cheese (cheddar, mozzarella)
- Optional: Sliced jalapeños, diced tomatoes

Instructions:
1. Heat a non-stick skillet over medium heat.
2. Place a tortilla in the skillet and sprinkle with shredded cheese.
3. Add optional jalapeños and tomatoes if desired.
4. Top with another tortilla and cook until cheese melts and tortillas are golden brown.
5. Cut into triangles and serve warm.

16. Deviled Eggs

Ingredients:
- 6 hard-boiled eggs
- 2 tbsp mayonnaise
- 1 tsp Dijon mustard
- Salt and pepper to taste
- Paprika for garnish
- Fresh parsley for garnish

Instructions:
1. Peel and halve the hard-boiled eggs. Remove the yolks and place them in a bowl.
2. Mash the yolks with mayonnaise, Dijon mustard, salt, and pepper until smooth.
3. Spoon or pipe the yolk mixture back into the egg whites.
4. Sprinkle with paprika and garnish with fresh parsley.
5. Serve immediately or refrigerate until ready to serve.

17. Cottage Cheese and Pineapple
Ingredients:
- 1 cup cottage cheese
- 1/2 cup pineapple chunks (fresh or canned)
- Fresh mint leaves for garnish

Instructions:
1. Spoon cottage cheese into a bowl.
2. Top with pineapple chunks.
3. Garnish with fresh mint leaves.
4. Serve immediately.

18. Almond Date Energy Balls
Ingredients:
- 1 cup almonds
- 1 cup Medjool dates, pitted
- 1/4 cup shredded coconut
- 1 tbsp cocoa powder
- 1 tsp vanilla extract

Instructions:
1. In a food processor, blend almonds until finely ground.
2. Add dates, shredded coconut, cocoa powder, and vanilla extract. Process until the mixture forms a sticky dough.
3. Roll the mixture into small balls.
4. Store in an airtight container in the refrigerator until ready to serve.

19. Shrimp Cocktail
Ingredients:
- 1 lb cooked shrimp, peeled and deveined
- Cocktail sauce
- Lemon wedges

Instructions:
1. Arrange cooked shrimp on a serving platter.

2. Serve with cocktail sauce and lemon wedges on the side.
3. Keep chilled until ready to serve.

20. Stuffed Mushrooms

Ingredients:
- 12 large mushrooms, stems removed
- 1/2 cup cream cheese, softened
- 1/4 cup grated Parmesan cheese
- 1 garlic clove, minced
- 1 tbsp fresh parsley, chopped
- Salt and pepper to taste

Instructions:
1. Preheat oven to 375°F (190°C).
2. In a bowl, mix cream cheese, Parmesan cheese, garlic, parsley, salt, and pepper.
3. Fill each mushroom cap with the cheese mixture.
4. Place stuffed mushrooms on a baking sheet.
5. Bake for 15-20 minutes or until mushrooms are tender and the filling is golden brown.
6. Serve warm.

6. Chapter 5: Lunch Recipes

1. Grilled Chicken and Quinoa Salad

Ingredients:
- 1 cup cooked quinoa
- 1 grilled chicken breast, sliced
- 1 cup mixed greens
- 1/2 cup cherry tomatoes, halved
- 1/4 cup cucumber, diced
- 1/4 cup feta cheese, crumbled
- 2 tbsp olive oil
- 1 tbsp lemon juice
- Salt and pepper to taste

Instructions:
1. In a large bowl, combine cooked quinoa, mixed greens, cherry tomatoes, cucumber, and feta cheese.
2. Top with sliced grilled chicken breast.
3. In a small bowl, whisk together olive oil, lemon juice, salt, and pepper.
4. Drizzle dressing over the salad and toss gently to combine.
5. Serve immediately.

2. Lentil and Vegetable Soup

Ingredients:
- 1 cup dried lentils, rinsed
- 1 onion, diced
- 2 carrots, diced
- 2 celery stalks, diced
- 3 garlic cloves, minced
- 1 can (14.5 oz) diced tomatoes
- 6 cups vegetable broth
- 1 tsp dried thyme
- 1 tsp dried oregano
- Salt and pepper to taste
- 2 cups spinach leaves

Instructions:
1. In a large pot, sauté onion, carrots, and celery over medium heat until softened.
2. Add garlic and cook for another minute.
3. Stir in lentils, diced tomatoes, vegetable broth, thyme, oregano, salt, and pepper.
4. Bring to a boil, then reduce heat and simmer for about 30 minutes, or until lentils are tender.
5. Stir in spinach leaves and cook until wilted.
6. Serve hot.

3. Turkey and Avocado Wrap
Ingredients:
- 1 whole wheat tortilla
- 4 slices of turkey breast
- 1/2 avocado, sliced
- 1/4 cup shredded lettuce
- 1/4 cup shredded carrots
- 1 tbsp mayonnaise or hummus
- Salt and pepper to taste

Instructions:
1. Lay the whole wheat tortilla flat and spread with mayonnaise or hummus.
2. Layer turkey breast, avocado slices, shredded lettuce, and shredded carrots on the tortilla.
3. Sprinkle with salt and pepper.
4. Roll up the tortilla tightly and slice in half.
5. Serve immediately.

4. Spinach and Feta Stuffed Peppers
Ingredients:
- 2 bell peppers, halved and seeded
- 1 cup cooked brown rice
- 1 cup fresh spinach, chopped
- 1/2 cup feta cheese, crumbled

- 1/4 cup diced tomatoes
- 1 tbsp olive oil
- Salt and pepper to taste

Instructions:
1. Preheat oven to 375°F (190°C).
2. In a large bowl, mix cooked brown rice, chopped spinach, feta cheese, diced tomatoes, olive oil, salt, and pepper.
3. Stuff each bell pepper half with the rice mixture.
4. Place stuffed peppers in a baking dish and cover with foil.
5. Bake for 25-30 minutes, or until peppers are tender.
6. Serve hot.

5. Salmon and Asparagus
Ingredients:
- 2 salmon fillets
- 1 bunch asparagus, trimmed
- 1 tbsp olive oil
- 1 lemon, sliced
- Salt and pepper to taste
- Fresh dill for garnish

Instructions:
1. Preheat oven to 400°F (200°C).
2. Place salmon fillets and asparagus on a baking sheet.
3. Drizzle with olive oil and season with salt and pepper.
4. Arrange lemon slices on top of the salmon.
5. Bake for 15-20 minutes, or until salmon is cooked through and asparagus is tender.
6. Garnish with fresh dill before serving.

6. Chickpea and Avocado Salad
Ingredients:
- 1 can (15 oz) chickpeas, drained and rinsed
- 1 avocado, diced

- 1/2 cup cherry tomatoes, halved
- 1/4 red onion, finely chopped
- 2 tbsp fresh parsley, chopped
- 2 tbsp olive oil
- 1 tbsp lemon juice
- Salt and pepper to taste

Instructions:
1. In a large bowl, combine chickpeas, avocado, cherry tomatoes, red onion, and parsley.
2. In a small bowl, whisk together olive oil, lemon juice, salt, and pepper.
3. Pour dressing over the salad and toss gently to combine.
4. Serve immediately or refrigerate until ready to serve.

7. Tuna and White Bean Salad
Ingredients:
- 1 can (5 oz) tuna in water, drained
- 1 can (15 oz) white beans, drained and rinsed
- 1/2 red bell pepper, diced
- 1/4 cup red onion, finely chopped
- 2 tbsp fresh basil, chopped
- 2 tbsp olive oil
- 1 tbsp red wine vinegar
- Salt and pepper to taste

Instructions:
1. In a large bowl, combine tuna, white beans, red bell pepper, red onion, and basil.
2. In a small bowl, whisk together olive oil, red wine vinegar, salt, and pepper.
3. Pour dressing over the salad and toss gently to combine.
4. Serve immediately or refrigerate until ready to serve.

8. Veggie-Packed Hummus Wrap
Ingredients:

- 1 whole wheat tortilla
- 1/2 cup hummus
- 1/4 cup shredded carrots
- 1/4 cup cucumber slices
- 1/4 cup red bell pepper strips
- Handful of spinach leaves
- 2 tbsp feta cheese, crumbled
- Salt and pepper to taste

Instructions:
1. Spread hummus evenly over the whole wheat tortilla.
2. Layer shredded carrots, cucumber slices, red bell pepper strips, spinach leaves, and feta cheese on the tortilla.
3. Sprinkle with salt and pepper.
4. Roll up the tortilla tightly and slice in half.
5. Serve immediately.

9. Baked Cod with Lemon and Herbs

Ingredients:
- 2 cod fillets
- 1 lemon, sliced
- 2 tbsp olive oil
- 2 tbsp fresh parsley, chopped
- 1 tsp dried thyme
- Salt and pepper to taste

Instructions:
1. Preheat oven to 375°F (190°C).
2. Place cod fillets in a baking dish.
3. Drizzle with olive oil and season with salt, pepper, and dried thyme.
4. Arrange lemon slices on top of the cod fillets.
5. Bake for 20-25 minutes, or until the fish is cooked through and flakes easily with a fork.
6. Garnish with fresh parsley before serving.

10. Quinoa Stuffed Tomatoes

Ingredients:
- 4 large tomatoes
- 1 cup cooked quinoa
- 1/2 cup spinach, chopped
- 1/4 cup feta cheese, crumbled
- 1/4 cup red onion, finely chopped
- 1 garlic clove, minced
- 2 tbsp olive oil
- Salt and pepper to taste

Instructions:
1. Preheat oven to 375°F (190°C).
2. Slice the tops off the tomatoes and scoop out the insides.
3. In a bowl, mix cooked quinoa, spinach, feta cheese, red onion, garlic, olive oil, salt, and pepper.
4. Stuff each tomato with the quinoa mixture.
5. Place stuffed tomatoes in a baking dish and cover with foil.
6. Bake for 20-25 minutes, or until tomatoes are tender.
7. Serve hot.

11. Chicken and Vegetable Stir-Fry

Ingredients:
- 1 lb boneless, skinless chicken breast, sliced
- 2 cups mixed vegetables (broccoli, bell peppers, snap peas)
- 2 garlic cloves, minced
- 1 tbsp fresh ginger, minced
- 2 tbsp soy sauce (low-sodium)
- 1 tbsp olive oil
- 1 tbsp sesame oil
- Cooked brown rice for serving

Instructions:
1. Heat olive oil in a large skillet over medium-high heat.
2. Add sliced chicken breast and cook until browned and cooked through.

3. Remove chicken from skillet and set aside.
4. In the same skillet, add mixed vegetables, garlic, and ginger. Cook until vegetables are tender-crisp.
5. Return chicken to the skillet and add soy sauce and sesame oil. Stir to combine.
6. Serve over cooked brown rice.

12. Mediterranean Chicken Pita
Ingredients:
- 1 whole wheat pita pocket
- 1 grilled chicken breast, sliced
- 1/4 cup hummus
- 1/4 cup diced cucumber
- 1/4 cup diced tomatoes
- 1/4 cup crumbled feta cheese
- Handful of mixed greens
- 1 tbsp olive oil
- 1 tsp lemon juice
- Salt and pepper to taste

Instructions:
1. Cut the pita pocket in half to create two pockets.
2. Spread hummus inside each pita pocket.
3. Fill with grilled chicken slices, diced cucumber, diced tomatoes, feta cheese, and mixed greens.
4. Drizzle with olive oil and lemon juice. Season with salt and pepper.
5. Serve immediately.

13. Turkey and Spinach Stuffed Sweet Potatoes
Ingredients:
- 2 large sweet potatoes
- 1/2 lb ground turkey
- 2 cups fresh spinach, chopped
- 1/2 cup diced tomatoes
- 1/4 cup shredded mozzarella cheese

- 1 tbsp olive oil
- 1 tsp garlic powder
- Salt and pepper to taste

Instructions:
1. Preheat oven to 400°F (200°C).
2. Wash sweet potatoes and pierce them several times with a fork. Bake for 45-50 minutes or until tender.
3. While sweet potatoes are baking, heat olive oil in a skillet over medium heat. Add ground turkey and cook until browned.
4. Add chopped spinach and diced tomatoes to the skillet. Cook until spinach is wilted and tomatoes are softened. Season with garlic powder, salt, and pepper.
5. Remove sweet potatoes from the oven and let cool slightly. Cut in half lengthwise and scoop out some of the flesh to create space for the filling.
6. Fill each sweet potato half with the turkey and spinach mixture. Top with shredded mozzarella cheese.
7. Return stuffed sweet potatoes to the oven and bake for an additional 10 minutes or until cheese is melted and bubbly.
8. Serve hot.

14. Greek Salad with Grilled Shrimp

Ingredients:
- 1 lb large shrimp, peeled and deveined
- 1 tbsp olive oil
- 1 tsp dried oregano
- Salt and pepper to taste
- 4 cups mixed greens
- 1/2 cup cherry tomatoes, halved
- 1/2 cucumber, sliced
- 1/4 red onion, thinly sliced
- 1/4 cup Kalamata olives
- 1/4 cup crumbled feta cheese
- 2 tbsp red wine vinegar

Instructions:
1. Preheat grill or grill pan over medium-high heat.
2. Toss shrimp with olive oil, dried oregano, salt, and pepper. Grill shrimp for 2-3 minutes on each side or until cooked through.
3. In a large bowl, combine mixed greens, cherry tomatoes, cucumber, red onion, olives, and feta cheese.
4. Top salad with grilled shrimp.
5. Drizzle with red wine vinegar and toss gently to combine.
6. Serve immediately.

15. Black Bean and Avocado Tacos

Ingredients:
- 1 can (15 oz) black beans, drained and rinsed
- 1 avocado, diced
- 1/2 cup corn kernels (fresh, frozen, or canned)
- 1/4 cup red onion, finely chopped
- 1/4 cup fresh cilantro, chopped
- Juice of 1 lime
- 1 tsp cumin
- 1 tsp chili powder
- Salt and pepper to taste
- 8 small corn tortillas

Instructions:
1. In a bowl, combine black beans, diced avocado, corn kernels, red onion, cilantro, lime juice, cumin, chili powder, salt, and pepper. Toss gently to combine.
2. Warm tortillas in a dry skillet over medium heat.
3. Spoon the black bean and avocado mixture onto each tortilla.
4. Serve immediately with additional lime wedges if desired.

16. Zucchini Noodles with Pesto and Cherry Tomatoes

Ingredients:
- 4 zucchinis, spiralized into noodles
- 1 cup cherry tomatoes, halved

- 1/4 cup pesto sauce (store-bought or homemade)
- 2 tbsp olive oil
- 2 tbsp grated Parmesan cheese
- Salt and pepper to taste

Instructions:
1. Heat olive oil in a large skillet over medium heat.
2. Add zucchini noodles and cook for 2-3 minutes until slightly softened.
3. Add cherry tomatoes and cook for another 2 minutes.
4. Remove from heat and stir in pesto sauce. Season with salt and pepper.
5. Top with grated Parmesan cheese before serving.

17. Eggplant Parmesan

Ingredients:
- 1 large eggplant, sliced into 1/2-inch rounds
- 1 cup marinara sauce
- 1 cup shredded mozzarella cheese
- 1/4 cup grated Parmesan cheese
- 1 tbsp olive oil
- 1 tsp dried basil
- Salt and pepper to taste

Instructions:
1. Preheat oven to 375°F (190°C).
2. Arrange eggplant slices on a baking sheet and brush with olive oil. Season with salt, pepper, and dried basil.
3. Bake for 20 minutes, flipping halfway through, until eggplant is tender and golden brown.
4. In a baking dish, layer eggplant slices, marinara sauce, and mozzarella cheese. Repeat layers, ending with a layer of mozzarella cheese.
5. Sprinkle grated Parmesan cheese on top.
6. Bake for an additional 20 minutes or until cheese is melted and bubbly.
7. Serve hot.

18. Chicken and Broccoli Stir-Fry

Ingredients:
- 1 lb boneless, skinless chicken breast, sliced
- 2 cups broccoli florets
- 1 red bell pepper, sliced
- 3 garlic cloves, minced
- 1 tbsp fresh ginger, minced
- 3 tbsp soy sauce (low-sodium)
- 1 tbsp sesame oil
- 1 tbsp olive oil
- Cooked brown rice for serving

Instructions:
1. Heat olive oil in a large skillet over medium-high heat.
2. Add sliced chicken breast and cook until browned and cooked through. Remove from skillet and set aside.
3. In the same skillet, add broccoli florets and red bell pepper. Cook until vegetables are tender-crisp.
4. Add garlic and ginger, cooking for another minute.
5. Return chicken to the skillet and add soy sauce and sesame oil. Stir to combine and heat through.
6. Serve over cooked brown rice.

19. Caprese Sandwich

Ingredients:
- 2 slices whole grain bread
- 1/2 cup fresh mozzarella, sliced
- 1 tomato, sliced
- Fresh basil leaves
- 1 tbsp balsamic glaze
- 1 tbsp olive oil
- Salt and pepper to taste

Instructions:
1. Toast the bread slices until golden brown.

2. Layer fresh mozzarella, tomato slices, and basil leaves on one slice of bread.
3. Drizzle with balsamic glaze and olive oil. Season with salt and pepper.
4. Top with the second slice of bread and serve immediately.

20. Beef and Vegetable Skewers

Ingredients:
- 1 lb beef sirloin, cut into cubes
- 1 red bell pepper, cut into squares
- 1 yellow bell pepper, cut into squares
- 1 zucchini, sliced into rounds
- 1 red onion, cut into squares
- 2 tbsp olive oil
- 1 tbsp soy sauce (low-sodium)
- 1 tsp dried rosemary
- Salt and pepper to taste

Instructions:
1. Preheat grill or grill pan over medium-high heat.
2. In a bowl, toss beef cubes, bell peppers, zucchini, and red onion with olive oil, soy sauce, dried rosemary, salt, and pepper.
3. Thread beef and vegetables onto skewers.
4. Grill skewers for 10-15 minutes, turning occasionally, until beef is cooked to desired doneness and vegetables are tender.
5. Serve immediately.

7. Chapter 6: Dinner Recipes

1. Lemon Herb Baked Salmon
- Ingredients:
  - 4 salmon fillets
  - 2 tablespoons olive oil
  - 2 cloves garlic, minced
  - 1 lemon (zested and juiced)
  - 1 teaspoon dried thyme
  - Salt and pepper to taste

- Instructions:
  1. Preheat oven to 400°F (200°C). Line a baking sheet with parchment paper.
  2. Place salmon fillets on the baking sheet. Drizzle with olive oil and lemon juice.
  3. Sprinkle minced garlic, lemon zest, thyme, salt, and pepper evenly over the fillets.
  4. Bake for 12-15 minutes, or until salmon flakes easily with a fork. Serve warm.

2. Quinoa-Stuffed Bell Peppers
- Ingredients:
  - 4 bell peppers, tops cut off and seeds removed
  - 1 cup quinoa, cooked
  - 1 cup black beans, drained and rinsed
  - 1 cup corn kernels
  - 1 cup diced tomatoes
  - 1 teaspoon cumin
  - 1/2 teaspoon chili powder
  - Salt and pepper to taste
  - 1/2 cup shredded cheddar cheese (optional)

- Instructions:
  1. Preheat oven to 375°F (190°C). Place bell peppers upright in a baking dish.
  2. In a bowl, combine cooked quinoa, black beans, corn, diced tomatoes, cumin, chili powder, salt, and pepper.
  3. Spoon quinoa mixture evenly into each bell pepper. Top with shredded cheese if desired.
  4. Cover with foil and bake for 25-30 minutes, or until peppers are tender. Remove foil and bake for an additional 5 minutes to melt cheese.

3. Mediterranean Chicken Skillet
- Ingredients:
  - 4 boneless, skinless chicken breasts
  - 1 tablespoon olive oil
  - 1 onion, diced
  - 2 cloves garlic, minced
  - 1 cup cherry tomatoes, halved
  - 1/2 cup Kalamata olives, pitted and sliced
  - 1/4 cup sun-dried tomatoes, chopped
  - 1 teaspoon dried oregano
  - Salt and pepper to taste
  - Fresh parsley for garnish

- Instructions:
  1. Season chicken breasts with salt, pepper, and dried oregano.
  2. Heat olive oil in a large skillet over medium heat. Add chicken and cook until browned and cooked through, about 6-8 minutes per side. Remove chicken and set aside.
  3. In the same skillet, add diced onion and cook until softened, about 3-4 minutes. Add minced garlic and cook for another minute.
  4. Stir in cherry tomatoes, Kalamata olives, and sun-dried tomatoes. Cook for 2-3 minutes until tomatoes are slightly softened.
  5. Return chicken breasts to the skillet. Cover and simmer for 5 minutes. Garnish with fresh parsley before serving.

4. Vegetarian Eggplant Parmesan
- Ingredients:
  - 2 large eggplants, sliced into 1/2-inch rounds
  - 2 cups marinara sauce
  - 1 cup shredded mozzarella cheese
  - 1/2 cup grated Parmesan cheese
  - 1/2 cup breadcrumbs
  - 2 tablespoons olive oil
  - Fresh basil leaves for garnish
  - Salt and pepper to taste

- Instructions:
  1. Preheat oven to 375°F (190°C). Lightly grease a baking sheet with olive oil.
  2. Arrange eggplant slices on the baking sheet. Brush both sides with olive oil and season with salt and pepper.
  3. Bake eggplant slices for 15-20 minutes, flipping halfway through, until tender and lightly browned.
  4. In a baking dish, spread a thin layer of marinara sauce. Layer half of the baked eggplant slices on top.
  5. Sprinkle half of the mozzarella and Parmesan cheese over the eggplant. Add another layer of marinara sauce, remaining eggplant slices, and top with remaining cheese.
  6. Sprinkle breadcrumbs evenly over the top. Bake for 20-25 minutes, until cheese is melted and bubbly.
  7. Garnish with fresh basil leaves before serving.

5. Lemon Garlic Herb Roast Chicken
- Ingredients:
  - 1 whole chicken (about 3-4 lbs)
  - 4 cloves garlic, minced
  - Zest and juice of 1 lemon
  - 2 tablespoons olive oil
  - 1 teaspoon dried thyme
  - 1 teaspoon dried rosemary

- Salt and pepper to taste

- Instructions:
  1. Preheat oven to 400°F (200°C). Rinse the chicken inside and out under cold running water, then pat dry with paper towels.
  2. In a small bowl, combine minced garlic, lemon zest, lemon juice, olive oil, thyme, rosemary, salt, and pepper.
  3. Rub the mixture evenly over the chicken, both inside the cavity and on the skin.
  4. Place the chicken breast-side up on a roasting pan or baking dish. Roast for 1 hour to 1 hour 15 minutes, or until the juices run clear and the internal temperature reaches 165°F (75°C).
  5. Let the chicken rest for 10-15 minutes before carving. Serve with roasted vegetables or a side salad.

6. Shrimp and Vegetable Stir-Fry
- Ingredients:
  - 1 lb shrimp, peeled and deveined
  - 2 cups broccoli florets
  - 1 red bell pepper, sliced
  - 1 cup snap peas
  - 1 carrot, thinly sliced
  - 2 cloves garlic, minced
  - 1 tablespoon ginger, minced
  - 1/4 cup low-sodium soy sauce
  - 2 tablespoons honey
  - 1 tablespoon sesame oil
  - Sesame seeds for garnish (optional)
  - Cooked brown rice or quinoa for serving

- Instructions:
  1. Heat sesame oil in a large skillet or wok over medium-high heat. Add minced garlic and ginger, and stir-fry for 1 minute until fragrant.
  2. Add shrimp to the skillet and cook until pink and opaque, about 2-3 minutes per side. Remove shrimp from skillet and set aside.

3. In the same skillet, add broccoli, bell pepper, snap peas, and carrot. Stir-fry for 3-4 minutes until vegetables are crisp-tender.

4. In a small bowl, whisk together soy sauce and honey. Pour over vegetables in the skillet and stir to combine.

5. Return cooked shrimp to the skillet and toss everything together until heated through.

6. Serve stir-fry over cooked brown rice or quinoa. Garnish with sesame seeds if desired.

7. Beef and Vegetable Stew
- Ingredients:
  - 1 lb stewing beef, cut into bite-sized pieces
  - 2 tablespoons olive oil
  - 1 onion, diced
  - 2 cloves garlic, minced
  - 2 carrots, peeled and chopped
  - 2 potatoes, peeled and diced
  - 1 cup green beans, trimmed and halved
  - 1 can (14 oz) diced tomatoes
  - 4 cups low-sodium beef broth
  - 1 teaspoon dried thyme
  - Salt and pepper to taste

- Instructions:
1. Heat olive oil in a large pot or Dutch oven over medium-high heat. Add stewing beef and cook until browned on all sides, about 5-7 minutes. Remove beef from pot and set aside.

2. In the same pot, add diced onion and cook until softened, about 3-4 minutes. Add minced garlic and cook for another minute.

3. Stir in carrots, potatoes, green beans, diced tomatoes (with juices), beef broth, dried thyme, salt, and pepper.

4. Bring stew to a boil, then reduce heat to low. Cover and simmer for 1.5 to 2 hours, stirring occasionally, until beef and vegetables are tender.

5. Adjust seasoning if needed before serving. Serve warm, garnished with fresh herbs if desired.

8. Vegetarian Lentil Curry
- Ingredients:
  - 1 cup dried lentils, rinsed
  - 1 onion, diced
  - 2 cloves garlic, minced
  - 1 tablespoon ginger, minced
  - 1 can (14 oz) diced tomatoes
  - 1 can (14 oz) coconut milk
  - 2 cups vegetable broth
  - 2 teaspoons curry powder
  - 1 teaspoon ground turmeric
  - 1 teaspoon ground cumin
  - Salt and pepper to taste
  - Fresh cilantro for garnish
  - Cooked rice or naan for serving

- Instructions:
  1. In a large pot, heat olive oil over medium heat. Add diced onion and cook until softened, about 3-4 minutes.
  2. Add minced garlic and ginger, and cook for another minute until fragrant.
  3. Stir in curry powder, turmeric, and cumin, and cook for 1 minute until spices are toasted.
  4. Add dried lentils, diced tomatoes (with juices), coconut milk, and vegetable broth to the pot. Season with salt and pepper.
  5. Bring mixture to a boil, then reduce heat to low. Cover and simmer for 25-30 minutes, or until lentils are tender and curry has thickened.
  6. Adjust seasoning if needed. Serve lentil curry over cooked rice or with naan bread. Garnish with fresh cilantro before serving.

9. Baked Stuffed Peppers with Ground Turkey
- Ingredients:
  - 4 bell peppers, tops cut off and seeds removed
  - 1 lb ground turkey
  - 1 onion, diced

- 2 cloves garlic, minced
  - 1 cup cooked quinoa
  - 1 cup marinara sauce
  - 1 cup shredded mozzarella cheese
  - Salt and pepper to taste
  - Fresh parsley for garnish

- Instructions:
  1. Preheat oven to 375°F (190°C). Place bell peppers upright in a baking dish.
  2. In a large skillet, cook ground turkey over medium heat until browned and cooked through, breaking it up with a spoon as it cooks.
  3. Add diced onion and minced garlic to the skillet with the turkey. Cook until onion is softened, about 3-4 minutes.
  4. Stir in cooked quinoa and marinara sauce. Season with salt and pepper to taste.
  5. Spoon turkey and quinoa mixture evenly into each bell pepper.
  6. Top each stuffed pepper with shredded mozzarella cheese.
  7. Cover with foil and bake for 25-30 minutes, or until peppers are tender and cheese is melted and bubbly.
  8. Garnish with fresh parsley before serving.

10. Ratatouille
- Ingredients:
  - 1 eggplant, diced
  - 2 zucchinis, diced
  - 1 yellow bell pepper, diced
  - 1 red bell pepper, diced
  - 1 onion, diced
  - 3 cloves garlic, minced
  - 1 can (14 oz) diced tomatoes
  - 2 tablespoons tomato paste
  - 1 teaspoon dried thyme
  - 1 teaspoon dried basil
  - Salt and pepper to taste

- Fresh basil leaves for garnish

- Instructions:
    1. Heat olive oil in a large skillet or Dutch oven over medium heat. Add diced eggplant and cook for 5-7 minutes, until softened.
    2. Add diced zucchini, bell peppers, and onion to the skillet. Cook for another 5 minutes, stirring occasionally.
    3. Stir in minced garlic, dried thyme, and dried basil. Cook for 1 minute until fragrant.
    4. Add diced tomatoes (with juices) and tomato paste to the skillet. Season with salt and pepper.
    5. Cover and simmer over low heat for 20-25 minutes, stirring occasionally, until vegetables are tender.
    6. Adjust seasoning if needed. Serve ratatouille warm, garnished with fresh basil leaves.

11. Mediterranean Stuffed Portobello Mushrooms
- Ingredients:
    - 4 large portobello mushrooms, stems removed
    - 1 cup quinoa, cooked
    - 1 cup cherry tomatoes, halved
    - 1/2 cup Kalamata olives, pitted and sliced
    - 1/2 cup crumbled feta cheese
    - 2 tablespoons olive oil
    - 2 cloves garlic, minced
    - 1 teaspoon dried oregano
    - Salt and pepper to taste
    - Fresh parsley for garnish

- Instructions:
    1. Preheat oven to 400°F (200°C). Place portobello mushrooms on a baking sheet, gill side up.
    2. In a bowl, combine cooked quinoa, cherry tomatoes, Kalamata olives, feta cheese, olive oil, minced garlic, dried oregano, salt, and pepper.
    3. Spoon quinoa mixture evenly into each portobello mushroom cap.

4. Bake for 15-20 minutes, until mushrooms are tender and filling is heated through.

5. Garnish with fresh parsley before serving.

12. Chicken and Vegetable Skewers with Tzatziki Sauce

- Ingredients:
  - 1 lb boneless, skinless chicken breasts, cut into cubes
  - 1 red bell pepper, cut into chunks
  - 1 yellow bell pepper, cut into chunks
  - 1 red onion, cut into chunks
  - 1 zucchini, sliced into rounds
  - 2 tablespoons olive oil
  - 2 cloves garlic, minced
  - 1 teaspoon dried oregano
  - Salt and pepper to taste
  - Wooden skewers, soaked in water

- Tzatziki Sauce:
  - 1 cup Greek yogurt
  - 1/2 cucumber, grated and excess water squeezed out
  - 1 clove garlic, minced
  - 1 tablespoon lemon juice
  - 1 tablespoon chopped fresh dill
  - Salt and pepper to taste

- Instructions:
  1. Preheat grill or grill pan over medium-high heat.
  2. In a bowl, combine olive oil, minced garlic, dried oregano, salt, and pepper. Add chicken cubes and vegetables, tossing to coat.
  3. Thread marinated chicken and vegetables onto skewers.
  4. Grill skewers for 8-10 minutes, turning occasionally, until chicken is cooked through and vegetables are tender.
  5. Meanwhile, prepare the tzatziki sauce by combining Greek yogurt, grated cucumber, minced garlic, lemon juice, chopped dill, salt, and pepper in a bowl. Mix well.

6. Serve chicken and vegetable skewers with tzatziki sauce on the side for dipping.

13. Spinach and Mushroom Stuffed Chicken Breast
- Ingredients:
  - 4 boneless, skinless chicken breasts
  - 1 cup spinach, chopped
  - 1 cup mushrooms, finely chopped
  - 1/2 cup ricotta cheese
  - 1/4 cup grated Parmesan cheese
  - 2 cloves garlic, minced
  - 1 tablespoon olive oil
  - Salt and pepper to taste
  - Toothpicks or kitchen twine

- Instructions:
  1. Preheat oven to 400°F (200°C). Line a baking sheet with parchment paper.
  2. In a skillet, heat olive oil over medium heat. Add minced garlic and cook for 1 minute until fragrant.
  3. Add chopped mushrooms and cook until softened, about 5 minutes. Stir in chopped spinach and cook for another 2-3 minutes until spinach wilts. Remove from heat.
  4. In a bowl, combine cooked spinach and mushrooms with ricotta cheese and grated Parmesan cheese. Season with salt and pepper.
  5. Butterfly each chicken breast by slicing horizontally through the middle, but not all the way through, to create a pocket.
  6. Stuff each chicken breast with the spinach and mushroom mixture. Secure with toothpicks or tie with kitchen twine to keep the filling inside.
  7. Place stuffed chicken breasts on the prepared baking sheet. Bake for 25-30 minutes, or until chicken is cooked through and juices run clear.
  8. Remove toothpicks or twine before serving.

14. Baked Salmon with Dill Sauce
- Ingredients:

- 4 salmon fillets
- 1 tablespoon olive oil
- Salt and pepper to taste
- Fresh dill sprigs for garnish

- Dill Sauce:
  - 1/2 cup Greek yogurt
  - 1 tablespoon Dijon mustard
  - 1 tablespoon lemon juice
  - 1 tablespoon chopped fresh dill
  - Salt and pepper to taste

- Instructions:
  1. Preheat oven to 400°F (200°C). Line a baking sheet with parchment paper.
  2. Place salmon fillets on the baking sheet. Drizzle with olive oil and season with salt and pepper.
  3. Bake salmon for 12-15 minutes, or until fish flakes easily with a fork.
  4. Meanwhile, prepare the dill sauce by combining Greek yogurt, Dijon mustard, lemon juice, chopped fresh dill, salt, and pepper in a bowl. Mix well.
  5. Serve baked salmon fillets with dill sauce drizzled over the top. Garnish with fresh dill sprigs.

15. Quinoa Stuffed Bell Peppers
- Ingredients:
  - 4 bell peppers, tops cut off and seeds removed
  - 1 cup quinoa, cooked
  - 1 can (15 oz) black beans, drained and rinsed
  - 1 cup corn kernels (fresh or frozen)
  - 1 cup cherry tomatoes, halved
  - 1/2 cup shredded cheddar cheese
  - 2 tablespoons olive oil
  - 2 cloves garlic, minced
  - 1 teaspoon ground cumin

- 1/2 teaspoon smoked paprika
- Salt and pepper to taste
- Fresh cilantro for garnish

- Instructions:
1. Preheat oven to 375°F (190°C). Place bell peppers upright in a baking dish.
2. In a skillet, heat olive oil over medium heat. Add minced garlic and cook for 1 minute until fragrant.
3. Stir in cooked quinoa, black beans, corn kernels, cherry tomatoes, ground cumin, smoked paprika, salt, and pepper. Cook for 3-4 minutes, stirring occasionally, until heated through.
4. Remove skillet from heat and stir in shredded cheddar cheese until melted and combined.
5. Spoon quinoa mixture evenly into each bell pepper.
6. Cover with foil and bake for 25-30 minutes, or until peppers are tender and filling is heated through.
7. Garnish with fresh cilantro before serving.

16. Vegetable and Chickpea Coconut Curry
- Ingredients:
  - 1 tablespoon coconut oil
  - 1 onion, diced
  - 2 cloves garlic, minced
  - 1 tablespoon grated ginger
  - 1 red bell pepper, diced
  - 1 yellow bell pepper, diced
  - 1 zucchini, diced
  - 1 can (15 oz) chickpeas, drained and rinsed
  - 1 can (14 oz) diced tomatoes
  - 1 can (14 oz) coconut milk
  - 2 teaspoons curry powder
  - 1 teaspoon ground turmeric
  - 1/2 teaspoon ground cinnamon
  - Salt and pepper to taste

- Fresh cilantro for garnish
   - Cooked rice or naan for serving

- Instructions:
   1. In a large pot or Dutch oven, heat coconut oil over medium heat. Add diced onion and cook until softened, about 3-4 minutes.
   2. Add minced garlic and grated ginger, and cook for another minute until fragrant.
   3. Stir in diced red bell pepper, yellow bell pepper, and zucchini. Cook for 5-7 minutes, until vegetables are slightly softened.
   4. Add chickpeas, diced tomatoes (with juices), coconut milk, curry powder, ground turmeric, ground cinnamon, salt, and pepper to the pot. Stir to combine.
   5. Bring curry to a boil, then reduce heat to low. Cover and simmer for 20-25 minutes, stirring occasionally, until vegetables are tender and flavors are blended.
   6. Adjust seasoning if needed. Serve vegetable and chickpea coconut curry over cooked rice or with naan bread. Garnish with fresh cilantro before serving.

17. Beef Stir-Fry with Vegetables
- Ingredients:
   - 1 lb flank steak, thinly sliced
   - 1 red bell pepper, thinly sliced
   - 1 yellow bell pepper, thinly sliced
   - 1 cup broccoli florets
   - 1 cup snow peas
   - 1 onion, thinly sliced
   - 2 cloves garlic, minced
   - 1 tablespoon ginger, minced
   - 1/4 cup low-sodium soy sauce
   - 2 tablespoons oyster sauce
   - 1 tablespoon sesame oil
   - 1 tablespoon cornstarch
   - 2 tablespoons water

- Cooked rice or noodles for serving

- Instructions:
   1. In a small bowl, whisk together soy sauce, oyster sauce, sesame oil, cornstarch, and water. Set aside.
   2. Heat a large skillet or wok over high heat. Add a drizzle of oil and stir-fry beef slices in batches until browned. Remove beef from skillet and set aside.
   3. In the same skillet, add a bit more oil if needed. Stir-fry minced garlic and ginger until fragrant, about 1 minute.
   4. Add sliced bell peppers, broccoli florets, snow peas, and onion to the skillet. Stir-fry for 3-4 minutes until vegetables are tender-crisp.
   5. Return cooked beef to the skillet. Pour the sauce mixture over the beef and vegetables. Stir-fry for another 1-2 minutes until sauce thickens and coats the beef and vegetables.
   6. Serve beef stir-fry immediately over cooked rice or noodles.

18. Spaghetti Squash with Turkey Meatballs
- Ingredients:
   - 1 medium spaghetti squash
   - 1 lb ground turkey
   - 1/2 cup breadcrumbs (gluten-free if desired)
   - 1/4 cup grated Parmesan cheese
   - 1 egg
   - 1 teaspoon dried oregano
   - 1 teaspoon dried basil
   - Salt and pepper to taste
   - 2 cups marinara sauce
   - Fresh basil leaves for garnish

- Instructions:
   1. Preheat oven to 400°F (200°C). Cut spaghetti squash in half lengthwise and scoop out the seeds.

2. Place squash halves cut side down on a baking sheet lined with parchment paper. Bake for 30-40 minutes, until squash is tender and can be easily pierced with a fork. Remove from oven and let cool slightly.

3. While squash is baking, prepare the turkey meatballs. In a bowl, combine ground turkey, breadcrumbs, grated Parmesan cheese, egg, dried oregano, dried basil, salt, and pepper. Mix until well combined.

4. Shape mixture into meatballs, about 1 inch in diameter.

5. In a large skillet, heat olive oil over medium heat. Add meatballs and cook until browned on all sides and cooked through, about 10-12 minutes.

6. Using a fork, scrape the spaghetti squash strands into a bowl.

7. Heat marinara sauce in a saucepan until warmed through.

8. To serve, place spaghetti squash strands on a plate, top with turkey meatballs, and spoon marinara sauce over the top. Garnish with fresh basil leaves.

19. Thai Peanut Chicken Stir-Fry
- Ingredients:
  - 1 lb boneless, skinless chicken breasts, thinly sliced
  - 1 red bell pepper, thinly sliced
  - 1 yellow bell pepper, thinly sliced
  - 1 cup snap peas
  - 1 carrot, julienned
  - 1/2 cup unsalted peanuts, chopped
  - 2 cloves garlic, minced
  - 1 tablespoon ginger, minced
  - 1/4 cup low-sodium soy sauce
  - 3 tablespoons creamy peanut butter
  - 2 tablespoons honey
  - 1 tablespoon rice vinegar
  - 1 teaspoon sesame oil
  - Cooked rice for serving

- Instructions:
  1. In a small bowl, whisk together soy sauce, peanut butter, honey, rice vinegar, and sesame oil. Set aside.

2. Heat a large skillet or wok over high heat. Add a drizzle of oil and stir-fry chicken slices until browned and cooked through. Remove chicken from skillet and set aside.

3. In the same skillet, add a bit more oil if needed. Stir-fry minced garlic and ginger until fragrant, about 1 minute.

4. Add sliced bell peppers, snap peas, julienned carrot, and chopped peanuts to the skillet. Stir-fry for 3-4 minutes until vegetables are tender-crisp.

5. Return cooked chicken to the skillet. Pour the peanut sauce mixture over the chicken and vegetables. Stir-fry for another 1-2 minutes until sauce coats everything evenly.

6. Serve Thai peanut chicken stir-fry immediately over cooked rice.

8. Chapter 7: Side Dishes

1. Garlic Roasted Brussels Sprouts

Ingredients:
- 1 lb Brussels sprouts, trimmed and halved
- 3 garlic cloves, minced
- 3 tbsp olive oil
- 1/2 tsp salt
- 1/4 tsp black pepper
- 1/4 cup grated Parmesan cheese (optional)

Instructions:
1. Preheat oven to 400°F (200°C).
2. In a large bowl, toss Brussels sprouts with garlic, olive oil, salt, and pepper.
3. Spread Brussels sprouts on a baking sheet in a single layer.
4. Roast for 20-25 minutes, or until Brussels sprouts are golden and tender, stirring halfway through.
5. Optional: Sprinkle with grated Parmesan cheese before serving.

2. Quinoa Salad with Cucumber and Mint

Ingredients:
- 1 cup quinoa, rinsed
- 2 cups water
- 1 cucumber, diced
- 1/4 cup fresh mint, chopped
- 1/4 cup red onion, finely chopped
- 2 tbsp olive oil
- 1 tbsp lemon juice
- Salt and pepper to taste

Instructions:
1. In a saucepan, bring quinoa and water to a boil. Reduce heat, cover, and simmer for 15 minutes, or until water is absorbed and quinoa is tender. Fluff with a fork and let cool.
2. In a large bowl, combine cooked quinoa, cucumber, mint, and red onion.
3. In a small bowl, whisk together olive oil, lemon juice, salt, and pepper.
4. Pour dressing over the quinoa salad and toss to combine.
5. Serve chilled or at room temperature.

3. Balsamic Glazed Carrots

Ingredients:
- 1 lb carrots, peeled and cut into sticks
- 2 tbsp olive oil
- 2 tbsp balsamic vinegar
- 1 tbsp honey
- 1 tsp dried thyme
- Salt and pepper to taste

Instructions:
1. Preheat oven to 400°F (200°C).
2. In a large bowl, toss carrots with olive oil, balsamic vinegar, honey, dried thyme, salt, and pepper.
3. Spread carrots on a baking sheet in a single layer.
4. Roast for 20-25 minutes, or until carrots are tender and caramelized, stirring halfway through.
5. Serve hot.

4. Steamed Broccoli with Lemon and Garlic

Ingredients:
- 1 large head of broccoli, cut into florets
- 2 garlic cloves, minced
- 2 tbsp olive oil
- Juice of 1 lemon
- Salt and pepper to taste

Instructions:
1. Steam broccoli florets in a steamer basket over boiling water for 5-7 minutes, or until tender but still crisp.
2. In a small skillet, heat olive oil over medium heat. Add garlic and sauté for 1-2 minutes, until fragrant.
3. Remove from heat and stir in lemon juice.
4. Toss steamed broccoli with the garlic-lemon mixture. Season with salt and pepper.
5. Serve immediately.

5. Sweet Potato Mash

Ingredients:
- 2 large sweet potatoes, peeled and cubed
- 1/4 cup milk (dairy or non-dairy)
- 2 tbsp butter or margarine
- 1/2 tsp ground cinnamon
- Salt and pepper to taste

Instructions:
1. Bring a large pot of water to a boil. Add sweet potato cubes and cook for 15-20 minutes, or until tender.
2. Drain and return sweet potatoes to the pot.
3. Add milk, butter, ground cinnamon, salt, and pepper.
4. Mash until smooth and creamy.
5. Serve hot.

6. Green Bean Almondine

Ingredients:
- 1 lb green beans, trimmed
- 2 tbsp butter or olive oil
- 1/4 cup sliced almonds
- 1 garlic clove, minced
- Juice of 1 lemon
- Salt and pepper to taste

Instructions:
1. Steam green beans in a steamer basket over boiling water for 5-7 minutes, or until tender-crisp.
2. In a large skillet, melt butter or heat olive oil over medium heat.
3. Add sliced almonds and garlic, and sauté until almonds are golden and garlic is fragrant.
4. Add green beans to the skillet and toss to coat.
5. Drizzle with lemon juice and season with salt and pepper.
6. Serve immediately.

7. Roasted Asparagus with Parmesan
Ingredients:
- 1 lb asparagus, trimmed
- 2 tbsp olive oil
- 1/4 cup grated Parmesan cheese
- Salt and pepper to taste

Instructions:
1. Preheat oven to 400°F (200°C).
2. In a large bowl, toss asparagus with olive oil, salt, and pepper.
3. Spread asparagus on a baking sheet in a single layer.
4. Roast for 12-15 minutes, or until asparagus is tender.
5. Sprinkle with grated Parmesan cheese before serving.

8. Cauliflower Rice
Ingredients:
- 1 large head of cauliflower, grated or processed into rice-sized pieces
- 2 tbsp olive oil
- 1 garlic clove, minced
- 1/4 cup fresh parsley, chopped
- Salt and pepper to taste

Instructions:
1. Heat olive oil in a large skillet over medium heat.
2. Add minced garlic and sauté for 1-2 minutes, until fragrant.

3. Add cauliflower rice and cook, stirring occasionally, for 5-7 minutes, until tender.
4. Stir in chopped parsley and season with salt and pepper.
5. Serve hot.

9. Greek Yogurt and Cucumber Salad

Ingredients:
- 1 cucumber, thinly sliced
- 1 cup Greek yogurt
- 1 garlic clove, minced
- 2 tbsp fresh dill, chopped
- Juice of 1 lemon
- Salt and pepper to taste

Instructions:
1. In a bowl, combine Greek yogurt, minced garlic, chopped dill, lemon juice, salt, and pepper.
2. Add cucumber slices and toss to coat.
3. Serve chilled.

10. Sautéed Spinach with Garlic and Lemon

Ingredients:
- 1 lb fresh spinach
- 2 tbsp olive oil
- 3 garlic cloves, minced
- Juice of 1 lemon
- Salt and pepper to taste

Instructions:
1. Heat olive oil in a large skillet over medium heat.
2. Add minced garlic and sauté for 1-2 minutes, until fragrant.
3. Add spinach and cook, stirring frequently, until wilted.
4. Remove from heat and stir in lemon juice.
5. Season with salt and pepper.
6. Serve immediately.

11. Herbed Couscous

Ingredients:
- 1 cup couscous
- 1 cup low-sodium vegetable broth
- 2 tbsp olive oil
- 1/4 cup fresh parsley, chopped
- 1/4 cup fresh mint, chopped
- 1/4 cup diced red onion
- Juice of 1 lemon
- Salt and pepper to taste

Instructions:
1. In a medium saucepan, bring vegetable broth to a boil.
2. Stir in couscous, cover, and remove from heat. Let stand for 5 minutes, or until liquid is absorbed.
3. Fluff couscous with a fork and transfer to a large bowl.
4. Stir in olive oil, parsley, mint, red onion, lemon juice, salt, and pepper.
5. Serve warm or at room temperature.

12. Garlic Mashed Cauliflower

Ingredients:
- 1 large head of cauliflower, cut into florets
- 3 garlic cloves, minced
- 1/4 cup milk (dairy or non-dairy)
- 2 tbsp butter or margarine
- Salt and pepper to taste
- Fresh chives, chopped (optional)

Instructions:
1. Steam cauliflower florets in a steamer basket over boiling water for 10-12 minutes, or until tender.
2. In a large bowl, combine steamed cauliflower, minced garlic, milk, and butter. Mash until smooth and creamy.
3. Season with salt and pepper.
4. Optional: Garnish with chopped fresh chives before serving.

- Side Dishes Recipes (Continued)

- 13. Roasted Beet and Goat Cheese Salad
- Ingredients:
- - 4 medium beets, scrubbed and trimmed
- - 2 tbsp olive oil
- - Salt and pepper to taste
- - 4 cups mixed greens
- - 1/4 cup crumbled goat cheese
- - 1/4 cup walnuts, toasted and chopped
- - 2 tbsp balsamic vinegar
- - 1 tbsp honey

- Instructions:
- 1. Preheat oven to 400°F (200°C).
- 2. Wrap each beet in aluminum foil and place on a baking sheet. Roast for 45-60 minutes, or until beets are tender.
- 3. Allow beets to cool slightly, then peel and cut into wedges.
- 4. In a large bowl, toss mixed greens with olive oil, balsamic vinegar, honey, salt, and pepper.
- 5. Top with roasted beets, crumbled goat cheese, and toasted walnuts.
- 6. Serve immediately.

- 14. Caprese Stuffed Portobello Mushrooms
- Ingredients:
- - 4 large portobello mushrooms, stems removed
- - 1 cup cherry tomatoes, halved
- - 1/2 cup fresh mozzarella, diced
- - 1/4 cup fresh basil, chopped
- - 2 tbsp olive oil
- - 1 tbsp balsamic glaze
- - Salt and pepper to taste

Instructions:
1. Preheat oven to 375°F (190°C).
2. Brush portobello mushrooms with olive oil and season with salt and pepper.
3. Place mushrooms on a baking sheet and bake for 15 minutes, or until tender.
4. In a small bowl, combine cherry tomatoes, fresh mozzarella, basil, salt, and pepper.
5. Fill each mushroom with the tomato mixture.
6. Drizzle with balsamic glaze before serving.

15. Lemon Dill Carrot Salad

Ingredients:
- 4 large carrots, grated
- 2 tbsp fresh dill, chopped
- 2 tbsp lemon juice
- 1 tbsp olive oil
- Salt and pepper to taste

Instructions:
1. In a large bowl, combine grated carrots, fresh dill, lemon juice, olive oil, salt, and pepper.
2. Toss to combine.
3. Serve chilled or at room temperature.

16. Broccoli Slaw with Apples and Cranberries

Ingredients:
- 4 cups broccoli slaw mix
- 1 apple, cored and diced
- 1/4 cup dried cranberries
- 1/4 cup slivered almonds
- 1/4 cup Greek yogurt
- 2 tbsp apple cider vinegar
- 1 tbsp honey
- Salt and pepper to taste

- Instructions:
- 1. In a large bowl, combine broccoli slaw, diced apple, dried cranberries, and slivered almonds.
- 2. In a small bowl, whisk together Greek yogurt, apple cider vinegar, honey, salt, and pepper.
- 3. Pour dressing over the slaw mixture and toss to coat.
- 4. Serve chilled.

- 17. Roasted Butternut Squash with Sage
- Ingredients:
  - 1 large butternut squash, peeled and cubed
  - 2 tbsp olive oil
  - 1 tsp dried sage
  - Salt and pepper to taste

- Instructions:
- 1. Preheat oven to 400°F (200°C).
- 2. In a large bowl, toss butternut squash cubes with olive oil, dried sage, salt, and pepper.
- 3. Spread squash on a baking sheet in a single layer.
- 4. Roast for 25-30 minutes, or until tender and caramelized, stirring halfway through.
- 5. Serve hot.

- 18. Cucumber and Tomato Salad with Feta
- Ingredients:
  - 2 cucumbers, diced
  - 2 cups cherry tomatoes, halved
  - 1/4 cup red onion, thinly sliced
  - 1/4 cup crumbled feta cheese
  - 2 tbsp olive oil
  - 1 tbsp red wine vinegar
  - Salt and pepper to taste

- Instructions:
- 1. In a large bowl, combine diced cucumbers, cherry tomatoes, red onion, and crumbled feta cheese.
- 2. In a small bowl, whisk together olive oil, red wine vinegar, salt, and pepper.
- 3. Pour dressing over the salad and toss to combine.
- 4. Serve chilled or at room temperature.
-
- 19. Garlic Sautéed Kale
- Ingredients:
- - 1 large bunch of kale, stems removed and leaves chopped
- - 3 garlic cloves, minced
- - 2 tbsp olive oil
- - 1 tbsp lemon juice
- - Salt and pepper to taste
-
- Instructions:
- 1. Heat olive oil in a large skillet over medium heat.
- 2. Add minced garlic and sauté for 1-2 minutes, until fragrant.
- 3. Add chopped kale and cook, stirring frequently, until wilted.
- 4. Remove from heat and stir in lemon juice.
- 5. Season with salt and pepper.
- 6. Serve immediately.
-
- 20. Mediterranean Chickpea Salad
- Ingredients:
- - 1 can (15 oz) chickpeas, drained and rinsed
- - 1 cup cherry tomatoes, halved
- - 1/2 cup cucumber, diced
- - 1/4 cup red onion, finely chopped
- - 1/4 cup Kalamata olives, sliced
- - 1/4 cup crumbled feta cheese
- - 2 tbsp olive oil
- - 1 tbsp red wine vinegar
- - 1 tsp dried oregano

- - Salt and pepper to taste
-
- Instructions:
- 1. In a large bowl, combine chickpeas, cherry tomatoes, cucumber, red onion, Kalamata olives, and crumbled feta cheese.
- 2. In a small bowl, whisk together olive oil, red wine vinegar, dried oregano, salt, and pepper.
- 3. Pour dressing over the salad and toss to combine.
- 4. Serve chilled or at room temperature.
-
- Additional Tips:
- - Color and Texture: Include a variety of colorful vegetables and different textures to make side dishes more appealing.
- - Make Ahead: Many side dishes can be prepared ahead of time and stored in the refrigerator, making meal prep easier.
- - Balanced Nutrition: Ensure side dishes complement the main meals by adding essential nutrients and balancing flavors.
-

9. Chapter 8: Desserts

1. Blueberry Chia Pudding
Ingredients:
- 1 cup unsweetened almond milk
- 1/2 cup fresh blueberries
- 3 tbsp chia seeds
- 1 tbsp maple syrup or honey
- 1/2 tsp vanilla extract

Instructions:
1. In a blender, combine almond milk, blueberries, maple syrup or honey, and vanilla extract. Blend until smooth.
2. Pour the mixture into a bowl and stir in chia seeds.
3. Cover and refrigerate for at least 4 hours or overnight, until the chia seeds have absorbed the liquid and the pudding has thickened.
4. Stir before serving. Garnish with additional blueberries if desired.

2. Baked Apples with Cinnamon and Walnuts
Ingredients:
- 4 medium apples
- 1/4 cup chopped walnuts
- 2 tbsp honey
- 1 tsp ground cinnamon
- 1/4 tsp ground nutmeg
- 1/4 cup water

Instructions:
1. Preheat oven to 375°F (190°C).
2. Core the apples and place them in a baking dish.
3. In a small bowl, combine chopped walnuts, honey, ground cinnamon, and ground nutmeg. Fill the center of each apple with the walnut mixture.
4. Pour water into the baking dish around the apples.
5. Bake for 30-40 minutes, or until apples are tender.

6. Serve warm, optionally with a dollop of Greek yogurt or a sprinkle of extra cinnamon.

3. Dark Chocolate Avocado Mousse

Ingredients:
- 2 ripe avocados, peeled and pitted
- 1/4 cup unsweetened cocoa powder
- 1/4 cup maple syrup or honey
- 1/4 cup unsweetened almond milk
- 1 tsp vanilla extract
- A pinch of salt

Instructions:
1. In a food processor or blender, combine avocados, cocoa powder, maple syrup or honey, almond milk, vanilla extract, and a pinch of salt.
2. Blend until smooth and creamy.
3. Spoon the mousse into serving bowls and refrigerate for at least 30 minutes before serving.
4. Garnish with fresh berries or a sprinkle of cocoa powder if desired.

4. Greek Yogurt Parfait with Berries

Ingredients:
- 2 cups Greek yogurt
- 1 cup mixed fresh berries (blueberries, strawberries, raspberries)
- 1/4 cup granola
- 2 tbsp honey
- 1 tsp vanilla extract

Instructions:
1. In a small bowl, mix Greek yogurt with honey and vanilla extract.
2. In serving glasses or bowls, layer Greek yogurt, mixed berries, and granola.
3. Repeat the layers until all ingredients are used, finishing with a layer of berries and granola.
4. Serve immediately or refrigerate for up to 2 hours.

5. Oatmeal Banana Cookies

Ingredients:
- 2 ripe bananas, mashed
- 1 cup rolled oats
- 1/4 cup raisins or chocolate chips
- 1/2 tsp ground cinnamon
- 1 tsp vanilla extract

Instructions:
1. Preheat oven to 350°F (175°C).
2. In a large bowl, combine mashed bananas, rolled oats, raisins or chocolate chips, ground cinnamon, and vanilla extract.
3. Drop spoonfuls of the mixture onto a baking sheet lined with parchment paper.
4. Flatten each cookie slightly with the back of a spoon.
5. Bake for 15-20 minutes, or until golden brown.
6. Allow cookies to cool on a wire rack before serving.

6. Strawberry Banana Nice Cream

Ingredients:
- 2 ripe bananas, sliced and frozen
- 1 cup strawberries, hulled and frozen
- 1/4 cup unsweetened almond milk
- 1 tsp vanilla extract

Instructions:
1. In a food processor or blender, combine frozen bananas, frozen strawberries, almond milk, and vanilla extract.
2. Blend until smooth and creamy, scraping down the sides as needed.
3. Serve immediately for a soft-serve consistency, or transfer to a container and freeze for 1-2 hours for a firmer texture.
4. Scoop into bowls and enjoy.

7. Apple Cinnamon Overnight Oats

Ingredients:

- 1/2 cup rolled oats
- 1/2 cup unsweetened almond milk
- 1/4 cup unsweetened applesauce
- 1/2 apple, diced
- 1/2 tsp ground cinnamon
- 1 tsp chia seeds (optional)
- 1 tsp honey or maple syrup (optional)

Instructions:
1. In a jar or container, combine rolled oats, almond milk, applesauce, diced apple, ground cinnamon, chia seeds, and honey or maple syrup if using.
2. Stir well to combine.
3. Cover and refrigerate overnight, or for at least 4 hours.
4. Stir before serving and enjoy cold.

8. Pumpkin Spice Energy Balls

Ingredients:
- 1 cup rolled oats
- 1/4 cup pumpkin puree
- 1/4 cup almond butter
- 2 tbsp honey or maple syrup
- 1 tsp ground cinnamon
- 1/2 tsp ground nutmeg
- 1/4 tsp ground ginger
- 1/4 cup mini chocolate chips (optional)

Instructions:
1. In a large bowl, combine rolled oats, pumpkin puree, almond butter, honey or maple syrup, ground cinnamon, ground nutmeg, and ground ginger.
2. Stir in mini chocolate chips if using.
3. Roll the mixture into small balls, about 1 inch in diameter.
4. Place the energy balls on a baking sheet lined with parchment paper and refrigerate for at least 30 minutes to firm up.
5. Store in an airtight container in the refrigerator for up to 1 week.

9. Baked Pears with Honey and Walnuts

Ingredients:
- 4 pears, halved and cored
- 1/4 cup walnuts, chopped
- 2 tbsp honey
- 1/2 tsp ground cinnamon
- 1/4 tsp ground nutmeg

Instructions:
1. Preheat oven to 350°F (175°C).
2. Place pear halves in a baking dish, cut side up.
3. In a small bowl, combine chopped walnuts, honey, ground cinnamon, and ground nutmeg.
4. Spoon the walnut mixture into the center of each pear half.
5. Bake for 20-25 minutes, or until pears are tender.
6. Serve warm, optionally with a scoop of Greek yogurt.

10. Coconut Mango Chia Pudding

Ingredients:
- 1 cup coconut milk
- 1/2 cup diced fresh mango
- 3 tbsp chia seeds
- 1 tbsp honey or maple syrup
- 1/2 tsp vanilla extract

Instructions:
1. In a blender, combine coconut milk, diced mango, honey or maple syrup, and vanilla extract. Blend until smooth.
2. Pour the mixture into a bowl and stir in chia seeds.
3. Cover and refrigerate for at least 4 hours or overnight, until the chia seeds have absorbed the liquid and the pudding has thickened.
4. Stir before serving. Garnish with additional mango if desired.

11. Almond Butter Banana Bites

Ingredients:
- 2 bananas, sliced into rounds
- 1/4 cup almond butter
- 1/4 cup dark chocolate chips, melted
- 1 tbsp coconut oil
- 1/4 cup crushed almonds

Instructions:
1. Spread a small amount of almond butter on half of the banana slices.
2. Top with the remaining banana slices to make little sandwiches.
3. In a microwave-safe bowl, combine dark chocolate chips and coconut oil. Microwave in 30-second intervals, stirring each time, until melted and smooth.
4. Dip each banana sandwich into the melted chocolate, then roll in crushed almonds.
5. Place the banana bites on a baking sheet lined with parchment paper and freeze for at least 1 hour.
6. Serve frozen for a refreshing treat.

12. Avocado Lime Cheesecake Bites

Ingredients:
- 1 cup almond flour
- 2 tbsp coconut oil, melted
- 2 ripe avocados, peeled and pitted
- 1/4 cup fresh lime juice
- 1/4 cup honey or maple syrup
- 1 tsp vanilla extract

Instructions:
1. In a small bowl, mix almond flour and melted coconut oil until combined. Press mixture into the bottom of a mini muffin tin to form the crust.
2. In a blender or food processor, combine avocados, lime juice, honey or maple syrup, and vanilla extract. Blend until smooth.
3. Spoon the avocado mixture on top of the crusts in the mini muffin tin.

4. Freeze for at least 2 hours, or until firm.
5. Serve frozen or slightly thawed.

13. Chia Seed Fruit Salad

Ingredients:
- 2 cups mixed fresh fruit (such as berries, kiwi, and mango)
- 2 tbsp chia seeds
- 1 tbsp fresh lime juice
- 1 tbsp honey or maple syrup
- Fresh mint leaves for garnish

Instructions:
1. In a large bowl, combine mixed fresh fruit, chia seeds, lime juice, and honey or maple syrup.
2. Toss gently to combine.
3. Let the salad sit for 10 minutes to allow the chia seeds to swell.
4. Garnish with fresh mint leaves before serving.

14. Cinnamon Baked Plantains

Ingredients:
- 2 ripe plantains, peeled and sliced into rounds
- 1 tbsp coconut oil, melted
- 1 tsp ground cinnamon
- 1 tbsp honey

Instructions:
1. Preheat oven to 375°F (190°C).
2. Place plantain slices on a baking sheet lined with parchment paper.
3. Brush the plantain slices with melted coconut oil.
4. Sprinkle with ground cinnamon and drizzle with honey.
5. Bake for 15-20 minutes, or until plantains are golden brown and caramelized.
6. Serve warm.

15. Yogurt and Berry Popsicles
Ingredients:
- 2 cups Greek yogurt
- 1 cup mixed fresh berries
- 2 tbsp honey or maple syrup
- 1 tsp vanilla extract

Instructions:
1. In a bowl, mix Greek yogurt, honey or maple syrup, and vanilla extract.
2. Layer Greek yogurt and mixed fresh berries in popsicle molds.
3. Insert popsicle sticks and freeze for at least 4 hours, or until fully frozen.
4. To release popsicles from the mold, run warm water over the outside for a few seconds.
5. Serve immediately.

16. Coconut Rice Pudding
Ingredients:
- 1 cup cooked jasmine rice
- 1 cup coconut milk
- 1/4 cup honey or maple syrup
- 1 tsp vanilla extract
- 1/4 tsp ground cinnamon
- 1/4 cup shredded coconut, toasted

Instructions:
1. In a medium saucepan, combine cooked jasmine rice, coconut milk, honey or maple syrup, vanilla extract, and ground cinnamon.
2. Cook over medium heat, stirring frequently, until the mixture thickens, about 10 minutes.
3. Remove from heat and let cool slightly.
4. Serve warm or chilled, topped with toasted shredded coconut.

17. Peach and Raspberry Crisp
Ingredients:
- 4 cups sliced peaches

- 1 cup raspberries
- 1/4 cup honey or maple syrup
- 1 tsp vanilla extract
- 1 cup rolled oats
- 1/2 cup almond flour
- 1/4 cup coconut oil, melted
- 1/2 tsp ground cinnamon

Instructions:
1. Preheat oven to 350°F (175°C).
2. In a large bowl, combine sliced peaches, raspberries, honey or maple syrup, and vanilla extract. Transfer to a baking dish.
3. In a separate bowl, mix rolled oats, almond flour, melted coconut oil, and ground cinnamon.
4. Sprinkle the oat mixture over the fruit.
5. Bake for 30-35 minutes, or until the topping is golden brown and the fruit is bubbly.
6. Serve warm, optionally with a scoop of vanilla ice cream.

18. Baked Cinnamon Pears

Ingredients:
- 4 ripe pears, halved and cored
- 1/4 cup walnuts, chopped
- 2 tbsp honey
- 1 tsp ground cinnamon

Instructions:
1. Preheat oven to 350°F (175°C).
2. Place pear halves in a baking dish, cut side up.
3. In a small bowl, combine chopped walnuts, honey, and ground cinnamon.
4. Spoon the walnut mixture into the center of each pear half.
5. Bake for 20-25 minutes, or until pears are tender.
6. Serve warm, optionally with a dollop of Greek yogurt.

19. Banana Oat Bars

Ingredients:
- 2 ripe bananas, mashed
- 1 1/2 cups rolled oats
- 1/4 cup almond butter
- 1/4 cup honey or maple syrup
- 1/2 tsp ground cinnamon

Instructions:
1. Preheat oven to 350°F (175°C).
2. In a large bowl, combine mashed bananas, rolled oats, almond butter, honey or maple syrup, and ground cinnamon.
3. Press the mixture into an 8x8-inch baking dish lined with parchment paper.
4. Bake for 20-25 minutes, or until the edges are golden brown.
5. Allow to cool before cutting into bars.

20. Pineapple Coconut Chia Pudding

Ingredients:
- 1 cup coconut milk
- 1/2 cup crushed pineapple, drained
- 3 tbsp chia seeds
- 1 tbsp honey or maple syrup
- 1/2 tsp vanilla extract

Instructions:
1. In a blender, combine coconut milk, crushed pineapple, honey or maple syrup, and vanilla extract. Blend until smooth.
2. Pour the mixture into a bowl and stir in chia seeds.
3. Cover and refrigerate for at least 4 hours or overnight, until the chia seeds have absorbed the liquid and the pudding has thickened.
4. Stir before serving. Garnish with additional pineapple if desired.

10. Chapter 9: Meal Plans

- 7-Day Meal Plan

Day 1: Monday

- Breakfast: Blueberry Chia Pudding
- Lunch: Chicken and Vegetable Stir-Fry with Brown Rice
- Dinner: Baked Salmon with Quinoa and Steamed Broccoli
- Snack: Greek Yogurt with Mixed Berries

Day 2: Tuesday

- Breakfast: Avocado Toast with Whole Grain Bread
- Lunch: Lentil Soup with a Side Salad
- Dinner: Turkey Meatballs with Zucchini Noodles
- Snack: Apple Slices with Almond Butter

Day 3: Wednesday

- Breakfast: Oatmeal Banana Cookies
- Lunch: Greek Salad with Grilled Chicken
- Dinner: Beef and Vegetable Stew with Mashed Cauliflower
- Snack: Carrot Sticks with Hummus

Day 4: Thursday

- Breakfast: Coconut Mango Chia Pudding
- Lunch: Quinoa Salad with Chickpeas and Roasted Vegetables
- Dinner: Baked Chicken with Sweet Potatoes and Asparagus
- Snack: Dark Chocolate Avocado Mousse

Day 5: Friday

- Breakfast: Greek Yogurt Parfait with Berries and Granola
- Lunch: Tuna Salad Lettuce Wraps
- Dinner: Baked Cod with Quinoa Pilaf and Green Beans
- Snack: Yogurt and Berry Popsicles

Day 6: Saturday

- Breakfast: Apple Cinnamon Overnight Oats
- Lunch: Caprese Salad with Grilled Shrimp
- Dinner: Eggplant Parmesan with Whole Wheat Pasta
- Snack: Cinnamon Baked Plantains

Day 7: Sunday

- Breakfast: Pumpkin Spice Energy Balls
- Lunch: Spinach and Mushroom Frittata
- Dinner: Vegetable Stir-Fry with Tofu and Brown Rice
- Snack: Chia Seed Fruit Salad

- Shopping Lists

Produce
- Fresh blueberries
- Fresh strawberries
- Fresh raspberries
- Fresh blackberries
- Fresh bananas
- Fresh apples (variety)
- Fresh pears
- Fresh peaches
- Fresh mango
- Fresh kiwi
- Fresh spinach
- Fresh kale
- Fresh broccoli
- Fresh asparagus
- Fresh green beans
- Fresh zucchini
- Fresh eggplant
- Fresh tomatoes
- Fresh cucumbers
- Fresh bell peppers (variety)
- Fresh carrots
- Fresh celery
- Fresh garlic
- Fresh ginger
- Fresh herbs (such as basil, mint, parsley)

Dairy & Eggs
- Greek yogurt (plain)
- Eggs
- Almond milk (unsweetened)

Protein
- Chicken breast
- Salmon fillets
- Cod fillets
- Ground turkey
- Tuna (canned or fresh)
- Tofu
- Shrimp

Grains & Legumes
- Rolled oats
- Brown rice
- Quinoa
- Whole grain bread
- Whole wheat pasta
- Lentils
- Chickpeas

Nuts & Seeds
- Chia seeds
- Almonds (whole or sliced)
- Walnuts

Pantry Staples
- Coconut oil
- Olive oil
- Honey or maple syrup
- Balsamic vinegar
- Soy sauce (low-sodium)
- Dijon mustard
- Canned crushed pineapple (in juice)
- Canned tomatoes (diced or crushed)
- Chicken or vegetable broth (low-sodium)
- Tomato paste

Frozen Foods
- Frozen mixed berries
- Frozen broccoli florets
- Frozen green peas

Snacks & Desserts
- Dark chocolate chips (semi-sweet or dark)
- Granola (preferably low-sugar)
- Hummus
- Whole grain crackers

Optional Ingredients (for specific recipes)
- Coconut milk (canned or carton)
- Avocado
- Nut butter (almond or peanut)
- Dark cocoa powder
- Raisins or chocolate chips
- Shredded coconut (unsweetened)
- Mini chocolate chips (dark or semi-sweet)

Beverages
- Herbal teas (various flavors)
- Sparkling water (plain or flavored)

Notes:
- Adjust quantities based on your specific needs and preferences.
- Check pantry items and spices to ensure you have enough of basics like salt, pepper, garlic powder, and other seasonings used in recipes.

This shopping list covers ingredients for a diverse range of meals including breakfasts, lunches, dinners, snacks, and desserts, ensuring you have everything you need to prepare nutritious and delicious meals throughout the week for seniors focusing on Alzheimer's and Dementia diet considerations.

- Tips for Meal Prep and Batch Cooking

Meal prep and batch cooking can significantly simplify meal times and ensure that seniors have nutritious options readily available. Here are some tips tailored for preparing meals from the Alzheimer's and Dementia diet cookbook for seniors:

Meal Prep Tips:

1. Plan Your Meals: Use the 7-day meal plan as a guide to plan your weekly meals. This helps streamline grocery shopping and ensures you have all ingredients on hand.

2. Prep Ingredients Ahead: Wash, chop, and portion out vegetables, fruits, and other ingredients needed for recipes. Store them in air-tight containers or zip-lock bags in the refrigerator for easy access.

3. Cook Grains and Proteins: Cook larger batches of brown rice, quinoa, chicken, and fish ahead of time. Store them in the refrigerator or freezer in portion-sized containers for quick assembly of meals.

4. Use Slow Cookers or Instant Pots: These appliances are great for batch cooking soups, stews, and casseroles. Set them up in the morning and have meals ready by dinner time.

5. Label and Date Containers: Clearly label containers with the name of the dish and date prepared. This helps keep track of freshness and ensures you're rotating through meals efficiently.

6. Portion Control: When portioning out meals, consider individual dietary needs and preferences. Some seniors may prefer smaller, more frequent meals while others may prefer larger portions less frequently.

Batch Cooking Tips:

1. Choose Freezer-Friendly Recipes: Select recipes that freeze well, such as soups, casseroles, and certain baked goods like muffins and cookies.

2. Invest in Freezer-Safe Containers: Use containers that are safe for freezing and can be easily reheated in the microwave or oven.

3. Cook in Bulk: Make double or triple batches of recipes when cooking. This saves time and effort in the long run and ensures you always have meals on hand.

4. Rotate Menu Items: Plan to rotate through a variety of dishes to keep meals interesting and ensure a balanced diet.

5. Consider Dietary Preferences: Tailor meals to individual tastes and dietary restrictions. Offer a variety of flavors and textures to keep meals enjoyable.

6. Reheat Safely: When reheating frozen meals, ensure they are heated thoroughly to the proper temperature to maintain food safety.

By implementing these meal prep and batch cooking tips, you can create a more efficient and enjoyable meal experience for seniors following the Alzheimer's and Dementia diet, ensuring they have nutritious and delicious meals readily available.

11. Chapter 10: Tips for a Healthy Lifestyle

- Incorporating Physical Activity

Incorporating physical activity into the daily routine of seniors following the Alzheimer's and Dementia diet is crucial for overall health and well-being. Here are some tailored tips to encourage and incorporate physical activity:

Types of Physical Activity:

1. Low-Impact Exercises: Focus on activities that are gentle on joints and muscles, such as walking, swimming, tai chi, or water aerobics. These can improve flexibility, balance, and cardiovascular health without causing strain.

2. Strength Training: Incorporate light resistance exercises using bands or light weights to maintain muscle strength. Simple exercises like arm curls, leg lifts, and seated squats can be beneficial.

3. Balance and Coordination Exercises: Practice exercises that improve balance and coordination, like standing on one foot, heel-to-toe walking, or using balance boards under supervision.

4. Stretching: Encourage gentle stretching exercises to improve flexibility and reduce stiffness. Yoga or seated stretching routines can be beneficial.

Tips for Incorporating Physical Activity:

1. Set Realistic Goals: Start with achievable goals based on the individual's fitness level and health condition. Gradually increase intensity and duration as tolerated.

2. Schedule Regular Activity: Establish a consistent schedule for physical activity, whether it's daily walks in the morning or participating in a senior fitness class a few times a week.

3. Make it Social: Encourage participation in group activities or exercises with family members or friends. Social interaction can enhance motivation and enjoyment.

4. Use Adaptive Equipment: Consider using walking aids or adaptive equipment to ensure safety and comfort during physical activity.

5. Modify Activities as Needed: Be flexible and modify activities based on individual abilities and preferences. Adapt exercises to accommodate any physical limitations.

6. Monitor Progress: Keep track of activity levels and progress to celebrate achievements and adjust goals as needed.

Safety Considerations:

- Consult with Healthcare Provider: Before starting any new exercise program, consult with a healthcare provider to ensure activities are safe and appropriate.

- Stay Hydrated: Encourage drinking water before, during, and after physical activity to prevent dehydration.

- Warm-Up and Cool Down: Incorporate gentle warm-up and cool-down exercises to prepare muscles and prevent injury.

By integrating these physical activity tips into the daily routine of seniors following the Alzheimer's and Dementia diet, you can promote overall health, enhance mood, and support cognitive function. Regular physical activity complements dietary efforts in maintaining a healthy lifestyle and improving quality of life.

- Importance of Social Engagement

Social engagement is crucial for seniors following the Alzheimer's and Dementia diet, as it plays a significant role in their overall well-being and quality of life. Here are key reasons why social engagement is important:

Cognitive Stimulation:

1. Enhances Cognitive Function: Social interactions stimulate the brain, promoting cognitive functions such as memory, problem-solving, and decision-making. Engaging in conversations and activities with others can help seniors stay mentally sharp.

2. Reduces Cognitive Decline: Studies suggest that active social engagement may help reduce the risk of cognitive decline and delay the onset of Alzheimer's disease and dementia. Social interactions challenge the brain and promote neuroplasticity.

Emotional Well-Being:

1. Reduces Feelings of Isolation: Social engagement provides opportunities for companionship and emotional support, reducing feelings of loneliness and isolation. Regular interactions with friends, family, and peers can uplift mood and reduce stress.

2. Promotes Positive Outlook: Being part of a social network can foster a sense of purpose and belonging, which contributes to overall emotional well-being. Positive social interactions can enhance self-esteem and confidence.

Physical Health:

1. Encourages Physical Activity: Social activities often involve physical movement and participation in group exercises or outings. Engaging in social activities can encourage seniors to stay physically active, improving cardiovascular health, muscle strength, and flexibility.

2. Supports Healthy Habits: Social networks can influence healthy lifestyle choices, including diet, exercise, and regular healthcare visits. Peer support and encouragement can motivate seniors to maintain healthy habits.

Mental Health:

1. Reduces Stress: Interacting with others and sharing experiences can provide emotional support and outlets for expressing feelings. Social engagement can buffer against stress and anxiety, promoting mental resilience.

2. Improves Mood: Regular social interactions can contribute to a positive mood and sense of happiness. Laughter, conversation, and shared activities can uplift spirits and improve overall mental health.

Tips for Promoting Social Engagement:

- Join Community Groups: Encourage participation in local senior centers, clubs, or hobby groups that align with interests.
- Attend Social Events: Encourage attending family gatherings, community events, or religious activities.
- Use Technology: Facilitate video calls or social media interactions with family and friends who may live far away.
- Volunteer: Engaging in volunteer work or mentoring programs can provide meaningful social connections and a sense of purpose.

- Stress Management Techniques

Managing stress is crucial for seniors following the Alzheimer's and Dementia diet to maintain overall well-being and cognitive health. Here are effective stress management techniques tailored for seniors:

Relaxation Techniques:

1. Deep Breathing: Encourage deep breathing exercises to promote relaxation. Inhale deeply through the nose, hold for a few seconds, and exhale slowly through the mouth. Repeat several times.

2. Progressive Muscle Relaxation: Guide seniors through tensing and relaxing each muscle group, starting from the toes up to the head. This technique helps release tension and promotes relaxation.

3. Guided Imagery: Use guided imagery scripts or recordings to help seniors visualize calming scenes or peaceful landscapes. This technique can reduce stress and promote a sense of calm.

Mindfulness and Meditation:

1. Mindfulness Practice: Teach seniors to focus on the present moment without judgment. Encourage mindful activities such as gentle yoga, walking meditation, or simply observing sensations, thoughts, and emotions.

2. Meditation: Introduce simple meditation practices focusing on breath awareness or repeating calming phrases (mantras). Regular meditation can reduce stress levels and enhance overall well-being.

Physical Activity:

1. Regular Exercise: Engage seniors in gentle physical activities such as walking, swimming, or chair exercises. Physical activity releases endorphins, which improve mood and reduce stress.

2. Tai Chi or Yoga: Encourage participation in tai chi or yoga classes designed for seniors. These practices combine gentle movements with deep breathing, promoting relaxation and stress reduction.

Social Support:

1. Maintain Social Connections: Foster regular social interactions with friends, family, or community groups. Sharing experiences and feelings with others can provide emotional support and reduce stress.

2. Join Support Groups: Recommend joining support groups specifically for individuals with Alzheimer's or dementia. These groups offer opportunities to share challenges and coping strategies with peers.

Healthy Lifestyle Choices:

1. Balanced Diet: Emphasize the importance of a nutritious diet rich in fruits, vegetables, whole grains, and lean proteins. A well-balanced diet supports overall health and resilience to stress.

2. Adequate Sleep: Encourage seniors to maintain a regular sleep schedule and practice good sleep hygiene. Sufficient sleep improves mood, cognitive function, and stress management.

Cognitive Stimulation:

1. Engage in Cognitive Activities: Recommend activities such as puzzles, crossword puzzles, reading, or learning new skills. Cognitive stimulation keeps the mind active and can reduce stress levels.

Environment and Routine:

1. Create a Calming Environment: Ensure the living space is comfortable, clutter-free, and promotes relaxation. Soft lighting, calming music, or nature sounds can contribute to a serene atmosphere.

2. Establish a Routine: Structure daily activities and meals around a consistent routine. Predictability and familiarity can reduce stress and anxiety for seniors.

Professional Support:

1. Consult Healthcare Providers: Encourage seniors to discuss stress management strategies with healthcare providers. They can provide personalized recommendations and support.

2. Counseling or Therapy: Consider counseling or therapy sessions if seniors experience persistent stress, anxiety, or depression. Professional support can help develop coping skills and emotional resilience.

By incorporating these stress management techniques into the daily routine of seniors following the Alzheimer's and Dementia diet, you can help them effectively manage stress, improve overall well-being, and enhance their quality of life. Regular practice of these techniques promotes resilience and supports cognitive health in the long term.

- Sleep Hygiene for Cognitive Health

Good sleep hygiene is essential for maintaining cognitive health, especially for seniors following the Alzheimer's and Dementia diet. Here are key practices to promote better sleep and support cognitive function:

Establish a Consistent Sleep Schedule:

1. Set a Routine: Encourage seniors to go to bed and wake up at the same time every day, even on weekends. Consistency helps regulate the body's internal clock and promotes better sleep quality.

2. Limit Daytime Naps: Discourage long or irregular daytime naps, as they can interfere with nighttime sleep. If necessary, encourage short, 20-30 minute naps earlier in the day to avoid disrupting sleep patterns.

Create a Comfortable Sleep Environment:

1. Optimize Bedroom Conditions: Ensure the bedroom is cool, quiet, and dark. Use blackout curtains or eye masks to block out light, and use earplugs or white noise machines to mask disruptive sounds.

2. Comfortable Bedding: Provide comfortable mattresses and pillows that support proper alignment and reduce discomfort during sleep.

Promote Relaxation Before Bed:

1. Establish a Bedtime Routine: Encourage seniors to wind down before bed with relaxing activities such as reading, listening to calming music, or taking a warm bath. A consistent bedtime routine signals to the body that it's time to sleep.

2. Limit Screen Time: Discourage the use of electronic devices (e.g., phones, tablets, TVs) close to bedtime, as the blue light emitted can interfere with the production of melatonin, a hormone that regulates sleep.

Encourage Healthy Lifestyle Choices:

1. Regular Exercise: Promote regular physical activity during the day, which can help seniors fall asleep faster and enjoy deeper sleep. However, avoid vigorous exercise close to bedtime, as it may be stimulating.

2. Dietary Considerations: Encourage a balanced diet that supports overall health and includes foods rich in sleep-promoting nutrients like tryptophan (found in turkey, nuts, and seeds) and magnesium (found in leafy greens, nuts, and whole grains).

Manage Stress and Anxiety:
1. Stress Reduction Techniques: Teach stress management techniques such as deep breathing, progressive muscle relaxation, or meditation to help

seniors relax before bedtime and reduce anxiety that may interfere with sleep.

2. Address Cognitive Stimulation: Engage in cognitive activities during the day to keep the mind active and promote mental relaxation before bed. Activities like puzzles, reading, or gentle hobbies can be beneficial.

Monitor and Adjust Sleep Habits:

1. Track Sleep Patterns: Encourage seniors to keep a sleep diary to monitor their sleep patterns, including bedtime routines, sleep duration, and any factors that may affect sleep quality.

2. Seek Professional Help if Needed: If seniors continue to experience sleep disturbances despite practicing good sleep hygiene, encourage them to consult healthcare providers. Sleep disorders or underlying medical conditions may require further evaluation and treatment.

By promoting good sleep hygiene practices tailored for cognitive health, you can help seniors following the Alzheimer's and Dementia diet improve sleep quality, support overall well-being, and enhance cognitive function over time. Regular, restorative sleep is crucial for memory consolidation, emotional regulation, and overall brain health.

12. Conclusion

In the journey towards supporting cognitive health through the Alzheimer's and Dementia diet, we embark not just on a path of nourishment, but on a profound commitment to enhancing quality of life and preserving cherished memories. Throughout this book, we've explored the intricacies of nutrition, the art of flavorful cooking, and the importance of holistic well-being for our beloved seniors.

Each recipe crafted with care is not just a meal but a testament to our dedication to their health. From the vibrant colors of antioxidant-rich berries to the comforting warmth of nutrient-dense soups, every ingredient has been chosen to nourish both body and mind. We've delved into the nuances of meal planning, encouraging routines that support stability and comfort, knowing that each bite can bring joy and sustenance.

Yet, beyond the recipes lies a deeper truth—that food is not merely sustenance but a bridge to connection. Whether shared around a table with family, prepared together with friends, or enjoyed in quiet moments of reflection, these meals foster bonds that transcend the kitchen. They are moments of laughter, of stories shared, and of love expressed through nourishing gestures.

As we navigate the complexities of Alzheimer's and Dementia, we acknowledge the challenges faced and the resilience shown every day. Through the principles of this diet, we strive not only to manage symptoms but to empower and uplift. We honor the courage of each individual and the unwavering support of caregivers, recognizing that together, we form a community bound by compassion and understanding.

In closing, let us continue this journey with compassion as our guide and nutrition as our ally. Let us savor each moment, knowing that through thoughtful choices and tender care, we can make a difference in the lives of those we cherish. May this book serve not only as a guide but as a source of inspiration—a reminder that every meal prepared with love is a gesture of hope, healing, and profound connection.

Together, let us embrace the nourishing power of food, the warmth of shared meals, and the enduring spirit that fuels our commitment to optimal health and well-being.

www.ingramcontent.com/pod-product-compliance
Lightning Source LLC
Chambersburg PA
CBHW082237220526
45479CB00005B/1259